'When people talk about sport competition they often enjoy those critical moments, fantastic performance, and unbelievable comeback in a final. They may well understand the philosophy of no pain, no gain, but in elite sport they still, however, underestimate how much pain those athletes stand in long term training. Tough training, high physical demand, and high pressure are often beyond the expectation or competence of athletes, and thus arouse mental health (MH) concerns from sport psychologists. As a book in the ISSP book series, *Mental Health in Elite Sport: Applied Perspectives from Across the Globe*, Professor Carsten Hvid Larsen, Karin Moesch, Natalie Durand-Bush, and Kristoffer Henriksen give us a good opportunity to have both an overall picture and a detailed view to understand how important MH is for athletes' sport career and long-term development. The discussions covered in this book include a variety of topics from conceptualization and definition of MH in elite sport to specific MH interventions across the globe. Those ideas and research findings about MH in elite sport are really very informative and inspiring for coaches, sport administration officers, athletes' parents, as well as applied psychology students and sport psychologists. I feel that it is also a must for those professionals and supporting team staff working within elite sports. Without understanding the psychological aspect of elite sport one can not understand elite sport as a whole. With the same reasoning, without understanding the MH of elite athletes one cannot understand elite athletes as a whole. So you are greatly encouraged to read this book. It is worth your time.'

Liwei Zhang, *Beijing Sport University, China*

MENTAL HEALTH IN ELITE SPORT

Mental Health in Elite Sport: Applied Perspectives from Across the Globe provides a focused, exhaustive overview of up-to-date mental health research, models, and approaches in elite sport to provide researchers, practitioners, coaches, and students with contemporary knowledge and strategies to address mental health in elite sport across a variety of contexts.

Mental Health in Elite Sport is divided into two main parts. The first part focuses globally on mental health service provision structures and cases specific to different world regions and countries. The second part focuses on specific mental health interventions across countries but also illustrates specific case studies and interventions as influenced by the local context and culture. This tour around the world offers readers an understanding of the massive global differences in mental health service provision within different situations and organizations. This is the first book of its kind in which highly experienced scholars and practitioners openly share their programs, methods, reflections, and failures on working with mental health in different contexts.

By using a global, multi-contextual analysis to address mental health in elite sport, this book is an essential text for practitioners such as researchers, coaches, athletes, as well as instructors and students across the sport science and mental health fields.

Carsten Hvid Larsen is an associate professor at the Faculty of Sport Science and Clinical Biomechanics at the University of Southern Denmark and head of sport psychology and sport psychology consultant in FC Nordsjaelland football club.

Karin Moesch is employed as a sport psychologist at the Department for Elite Sports at the Swedish Sports Confederation. She also holds a position as a researcher at the Department of Psychology at Lund University.

Natalie Durand-Bush is a sport psychology professor, scientist, and practitioner in the School of Human Kinetics at the University of Ottawa in Ottawa, Canada. Natalie is the Director of the SEWP LAB and the co-founder of the Canadian Centre for Mental Health and Sport (CCMHS).

Kristoffer Henriksen is an associate professor at the Faculty of Sport Science and Clinical Biomechanics at the University of Southern Denmark and sport psychology practitioner in Team Denmark.

INTERNATIONAL PERSPECTIVES ON KEY ISSUES IN SPORT AND EXERCISE PSYCHOLOGY

Series Editors
Robert J. Schinke
Thomas Schack
Athanasios Papaioannou

International Perspectives on Key Issues in Sport and Exercise Psychology is a series of edited books published in partnership with the International Society of Sport Psychology. Each title reflects cutting edge research in the psychological study of high level sport, written by key researchers and leading figures in the field of sports psychology.

Routledge Companion to Sport and Exercise Psychology
Global Perspectives and Fundamental Concepts
Edited by Athanasios Papaioannou and Dieter Hackfort

The Psychology of Sub-Culture in Sport and Physical Activity
Critical Perspectives
Edited by Robert J. Schinke and Kerry R. McGannon

Psychology in Professional Sports and the Performing Arts
Challenges and Strategies
Edited by Robert J. Schinke and Dieter Hackfort

Encyclopedia of Sport and Exercise Psychology
Volume 1: Theoretical and Methodological Concepts
Edited by Dieter Hackfort and Robert J. Schinke

Encyclopedia of Sport and Exercise Psychology
Volume 2: Applied and Practical Measures
Edited by Dieter Hackfort and Robert J. Schinke

Advancements in Mental Skills Training
Edited by Maurizio Bertollo, Edson Filho and Peter C. Terry

Mental Health in Elite Sport
Applied Perspectives from Across the Globe
Edited by Carsten Hvid Larsen, Karin Moesch, Natalie Durand-Bush, and Kristoffer Henriksen

For more information about this series, please visit: www.routledge.com/ISSP-Key-Issues-in-Sport-and-Exercise-Psychology/book-series/KISEP

MENTAL HEALTH IN ELITE SPORT

Applied Perspectives from Across the Globe

Edited by Carsten Hvid Larsen, Karin Moesch, Natalie Durand-Bush, and Kristoffer Henriksen

Routledge
Taylor & Francis Group
LONDON AND NEW YORK

First published 2021
by Routledge
2 Park Square, Milton Park, Abingdon, Oxon OX14 4RN

and by Routledge
605 Third Avenue, New York, NY 10158

Routledge is an imprint of the Taylor & Francis Group, an informa business

British Library Cataloguing-in-Publication Data
A catalogue record for this book is available from the British Library

Library of Congress Cataloging-in-Publication Data
Names: Larsen, Carsten Hvid, editor.
Title: Mental health in elite sport : applied perspectives from across the globe / edited by Carsten Hvid Larsen, Karin Moesch, Natalie Durand-Bush, Kristoffer Henriksen.
Description: Abingdon, Oxon ; New York, NY : Routledge, 2021. |
Includes bibliographical references and index. Identifiers: LCCN 2020054096 |
ISBN 9780367427672 (hardback) | ISBN 9780367427689 (paperback) |
ISBN 9780367854973 (ebook)
Subjects: LCSH: Professional athletes–Mental health. | Olympic athletes–Mental health.
Classification: LCC RC451.4.A83 M46 2021 | DDC 616.890088796–dc23
LC record available at https://lccn.loc.gov/2020054096

ISBN: 978-0-367-42767-2 (hbk)
ISBN: 978-0-367-42768-9 (pbk)
ISBN: 978-0-367-85497-3 (ebk)

Typeset in Bembo
by Newgen Publishing UK

CONTENTS

CONTRIBUTORS

Editors

Natalie Durand-Bush, Ph.D. is a sport psychology professor, scientist, and practitioner in the School of Human Kinetics at the University of Ottawa in Ottawa, Canada. Her areas of specialization include psychological skills training and assessment, mental health, and coaching psychology. Natalie is the Director of the SEWP LAB and the co-founder of the Canadian Centre for Mental Health and Sport (CCMHS) – a specialized Centre off ering collaborative sport-focused mental health care services to high-performance athletes and coaches. As a mental performance consultant for the past 25 years, Natalie has helped amateur and professional athletes and coaches of all ages, sports, and levels achieve their performance and well-being goals. A relentless advocate for the fi eld of sport psychology, she has co-founded and chaired the Canadian Sport Psychology Association (CSPA) and has served as the Vice-President of the International Society of Sport Psychology (ISSP). Natalie is currently the Past President of the Association for Applied Sport Psychology (AASP) and is an AASP Fellow. She is co-editing AASP's forthcoming *Essential Guide for Mental Performance Consultants*.

Kristoffer Henriksen, Ph.D. is an associate professor at the Institute of Sport Science and Clinical Biomechanics at the University of Southern Denmark. His research mainly looks at social relations and their infl uence on athlete development and performance with an emphasis on successful sporting environments. Since 2008 his employment has included a specialized function as a sport psychology practitioner in Team Denmark, corresponding to 50% of a fulltime position. In this function he has worked to develop high performance cultures in national teams and mentally strong athletes and coaches. He has worked in several sports, but mainly in orienteering and Olympic sailing and supported athletes and teams during several World Championships and during the London and Rio Olympic Games.

Carsten Hvid Larsen, Ph.D. is an Associate Professor at the Institute of Sport Science and Clinical Biomechanics at the University of Southern Denmark and head of sport psychology and sport psychology consultant in FCN football club. Since 2013 he has worked as a sport psychology consultant corresponding to 50% of a full-time position. His employment at FCN includes support for professional football players at the first team and under-19 team and moreover he supports the youth national teams in football (soccer). Previously he has supported athletes at the European, World Championships and the Olympic Games with a focus on team development, performance enhancement and developing resilient athletes and coaches.

Karin Moesch, Ph.D. is employed as a sport psychologist at the Department for Elite Sports at the Swedish Sports Confederation. In this position, she provides individual counseling, group workshops and educations for elite athletes and coaches, as well as therapy for elite athletes and coaches in the Clinic for Mental Health in Elite Sports in Malmö. Karin also holds a position as a researcher at the Department of Psychology at Lund University. Her research interests include psychological aspects of injury, mental health in elite athletes, team sports, and talent development. Since 2015, she has been a member of the managing council of the European Federation of Sport Psychology (FEPSAC), and is designated vice-president for the period 2019–2022.

Authors

Johanna Belz, Ph.D. is a researcher and lecturer at the German Sport University Cologne and is also working as a sport psychology consultant. She has degrees in both psychology (diploma) and sport science (M.Sc.). The main topics of her research are stress and mental health in elite athletes. She coordinates the German initiative *mentaltalent.de* at the German Sport University Cologne, providing sport psychological support for adolescent elite athletes in North Rhine-Westphalia.

Matt Butterworth is the Mental Health Manager at the Australian Institute of Sport. He has been a Clinical Psychologist since 2004 and has worked in child and adolescent, adult mental health, forensic and high-performance sports settings. He has worked in New Zealand, the UK, and Australia. Matt values the different perspectives and experiences that people bring having grown up in an environment that encapsulated both his NZ Maori and NZ European ancestry and cultures. He is passionate about helping people to lead their best life and continues to value all of the great things that sports involvement can bring to people, families, and communities: including better health, social connection, working and achieving together.

Cristina Carvalho de Melo graduated in Physical Education and Administration; Specialist in Sport Psychology; Master in Leisure, MBA in Project Management, Ph.D. student in Sports Science (UFMG). Professor of Sport Psychology at Centro Universitário UNA. Collaborating member of the ISSP Emerging Countries Project. Mental preparation of Minas Quad Rugby Team – four times national champion, Paralympic rugby.

Sarah Cecil is a Chartered Sport Psychologist and has 20 years of experience predominantly in Olympic and Paralympic sport. She supported the British Athletics team at London 2012. Post 2012 she worked at the Team GB Intensive Rehabilitation Unit for five years. Sarah was the sport psychologist for the UK Team at four Invictus Games from London to Sydney. Sarah sits on the UK Sport Mental Health Steering Group. She currently works with Wheelchair

Tennis and GB Snowsport. Sarah uses the expertise she has to enable athletes to deliver under pressure and to support coaches and performance staff to fulfil their potential.

Matti Clements is the Director, People Development & Wellbeing at the Australian Institute of Sport (AIS). Matti has over 15 years' experience working with Australia's top elite and professional sports at both a strategic and operational level. A qualified psychologist she has a broad expertise in the design, implementation, and ongoing management of national programs in the area of well-being, professional development services and support systems for high performance sporting organizations, which has included several AFL Clubs, Cricket Australia, Golf Australia, Netball Australia, Tennis Australia, AFL and the Australian Cricketers Association. Previously Matti was National Manager at the AFL Players Association, leading and developing the national well-being and life skills program to become an industry benchmark across Australia and internationally.

Alexander Cohen was appointed Senior Sport Psychologist at the U.S. Olympic & Paralympic Committee in 2011. Working primarily with winter sports, Dr. Cohen provides sport psychology consultation and counseling for national teams, athletes, and coaches at the Olympic Training Centers, at various National Governing Body training sites and at national and international competitions. As a licensed psychologist and certified sport psychology consultant, Dr. Cohen assists coaches in creating mastery performance environments that promote psychological and physical skill acquisition and execution. He works directly with athletes to maximize performance readiness through consistent preparation, enhanced resilience, and mindful self-regulation, helping athletes to focus on the right things, at the right time, every time. Dr. Cohen earned his bachelor's degree in psychology from Texas A&M, and later completed his master's in sport psychology and Ph.D. in counseling psychology from Florida State University. He completed a pre-doctoral internship with a specialization in sport psychology at Kansas State University, and a post-doctoral fellowship specializing in sport psychology at the University of Georgia.

Samuel Cumming is the Mental Health Manager at the English Institute of Sport (EIS) where he supports delivery of UK Sport's Mental Health Strategy across Olympic and Paralympic sports. His training is in psychology (B.Sc. in Applied Social Psychology with Clinical Psychology; M.Sc. in Sport Psychology) and before moving to the EIS in 2019 Sam worked with British Rowing in the management and support of the GB Rowing Team.

Marcelo Callegari Zanetti, Ph.D. graduated in Physical Education, and has a Master's degree in Human Motricity Sciences and Ph.D. in Human Development and Technologies. He completed a doctoral internship with a PDSE / CAPES scholarship at the Department of Psychology at the University of Québecà Trois-Rivières (Canada). He is Professor of Health Undergraduate courses at Paulista University in São José do Rio Pardo; Professor of the Undergraduate and the Graduate Program in Physical Education (Master and Ph.D.) at São Judas University in São Paulo. He qualified as an Empowering Coaching ™ Tutor at the Sport Psychology Research Unit at the Valencia University, Spain.

Justice Dipeba is a Sport Officer and an elite Coach in the Department of Culture, Sport & Recreation at the University of Botswana. He is also a retired athlete who represented Botswana at major international games including the 1996 Olympics in Atlanta, USA. He holds a Bachelor of Science in Education, (Physical Education) from Auburn University, (USA). He has been a Senior National Athletics Coach for more than ten years, specializing in sprints, relays, and hurdles. He has coached some of the most accomplished athletes including Isaac Makwala and Christine Botlogetswe.

Maria Regina Ferreira Brandão is a psychologist, postgraduate degree in Sports Psychology at the Higher Institute of Physical Culture of Havana, Cuba. She has a Master's degree in Human Development, a Doctorate in Sports Sciences and a Post-doctorate in Sports Psychology at FMH, Lisbon, Portugal. She is currently a professor of the Master's and Doctorate Program in Physical Education at the São Judas Tadeu University in Sao Paulo, Brazil; vice-president of the Iberoamerican Society of Sports Psychology (SIPD); member of the Brazilian Paralympic Academy and the Brazilian Academy of Coaches of the Brazilian Olympic Committee. She qualified as an Empowering Coaching™ Tutor at the Sport Psychology Research Unit at the Valencia University, Spain. She has had practical experience with mental preparation of Olympic athletes since Barcelona 92 and was past president of the Brazilian Association of Studies in Sports and Exercise Psychology (ABEPEEx).

Amanda Gatherer is a Consultant Clinical Psychologist, currently Chief Psychologist at Birmingham and Solihull Mental Health NHS Foundation Trust. She has extensive experience with elite athletes through her previous consultancy work with the England & Wales Cricket Board, as a Member of the EIS Mental Health Expert Panel and as Mental Health Lead for Paralympics GB.

Karin Hyland works as a senior consultant in psychiatry and was part of the team establishing the Mental Health Clinic for Elite Sports, Stockholm Centre for Dependence Disorders in Stockholm in 2015. She is also involved in the alcohol research field at the Department of Clinical Neuroscience, Karolinska Institutet. Karin has a broad experience from psychiatry and addiction where she has been active since 2002.

Göran Kenttä, Ph.D. earned his doctorate in psychology at Stockholm University in 2001. The majority of his research has focused on elite sports with a stress–recovery perspective. He currently holds a research position in Stockholm at The Swedish School of Sport and Health Sciences, and has been a director of the Coach Education Program at the university; he is also the past president of the Swedish Sport Psychological Association. In addition, Göran currently holds a position at the Swedish Sport Federation as Head of Discipline in sport psychology and an adjunct professor position at Ottawa University.

Jens Kleinert, Ph.D. is full Professor for Sport Psychology and Health Psychology at the Institute of Psychology at the German Sport University Cologne. He is Sport Scientist (diploma) and Physician (MD) and was both athlete and coach in swimming and handball. Currently, his lab group focuses on interpersonal relation in sport and exercise and its impact on motivation, mental health, and performance.

Andreas Küttel, Ph.D. is an Assistant Professor at the Institute of Sports Sciences and Clinical Biomechanics at the University of Southern Denmark. As a former elite athlete representing Switzerland in several Olympics and World Championships as a ski jumper, he has gathered first-hand experience about the dynamic state of mental health in high-performance sports.

His research interests are athletes' transitions and (dual) career with a focus on mental health. Since 2017, he supports the Swiss ski jumping national team as a sport psychological consultant applying a holistic approach on athletes' development in sport and life.

Frank J. H. Lu, Ph.D. is a Professor and Director at the Graduate Institute of Sport Coaching Science, Chinese Culture University, Taiwan. He is currently Vice President of the Asian-South Pacific Association of Sport Psychology (ASPASP). His major research in applied practices is the Psychology of Sport Excellence; specifically the Athletic Mental Energy (Lu et al., 2018,[1] Chiu et al., 2020[2]). He expects to expand athletic mental energy both in academic and applied sport psychology. By doing so, he hopes to enhance athletes' performance and well-being.

Lingani Mbakile-Mahlanza, Ph.D. is an Atlantic Senior Fellow with the Global Brain Health Institute. She holds a Doctorate in Clinical Neuropsychology and a Master's in Clinical Psychology. Dr. Mbakile-Mahlanza has an appointment at the University of Botswana as a lecturer (Assistant Professor) in the psychology department and as coordinator of the psychology clinic. She has a special interest in neurodegenerative conditions and traumatic brain injury. In addition to training psychologists and working clinically, she has been conducting research in the areas of mental health, dementia, traumatic brain injury, and neuropsychology in under-resourced settings.

Franco Noce, Ph.D. graduated in Physical Education and Psychology. Master's degree in Physical Education at the Federal University of Minas Gerais (UFMG), Ph.D. in Psychobiology at Federal University of Sao Paulo (UNIFESP). He is currently Adjunct Professor at the School of Physical Education (UFMG). He is a professor in the Sports Science Program/UFMG. Coordinator of Sector of Sport Psychology at Sports Center Training UFMG; ISSP Managing Council member since 2013; Chair of ISSP Emerging Countries Projects; and Vice President of the Brazilian Association of Studies in Sports and Exercise Psychology (ABEPEEx). He has had practical experience with mental preparation highlighting Paralympic Games in Athens (2004), Beijing (2008), and Rio (2016).

Gaorekwe V. Nthutang is the Deputy Director at the University of Botswana Student Affairs Division. She has vast experience in teaching, counseling, and protocol. She is a member of Botswana Health Professional Council, Botswana Association of Psychologists, Association of Applied Sports Psychology and is currently reading for a Ph.D. in Sport Psychology. She has consulted with a number of team (athletes and officials) at major games including Gaborone Youth Games, Netball World Youth Cup Tournament, Botswana Games, Confederation of University and Colleges Sports Association Games, Botswana Karate Association, and Region 5 Youth Games.

Lisa Olive is the recipient of an NHMRC Early Career Fellowship and Senior Research Fellow at the Centre of Social and Early Emotional Development (SEED), School of Psychology and at the Institute for Mental and Physical Health and Clinical Translation (IMPACT), School of Medicine, Deakin University. She is also an Honorary Senior Research Fellow at Orygen in the Elite Sport Unit, University of Melbourne. Lisa is a Clinical Psychologist with experience in clinical and sport settings, including previous roles at the Australian Institute of Sport and ACT Academy of Sport. She currently maintains a clinical private practice alongside her research work.

Rosemary Purcell is the Director of Research & Translation at Orygen and Associate Professor and Deputy Head of Department for the Centre for Youth Mental Health at The University of Melbourne. She is a registered psychologist and leads the Elite Sports and Mental Health program at Orygen. Rosie's research focuses on understanding the prevalence and nature of mental health problems in high performance sport, and optimal strategies for improving and maximizing mental health and well-being in elite sporting environments. She is interested in whole of organization ('systems') approaches to improving mental health in sport and has worked with a number of elite and professional sports in Australia to support their work in developing early intervention frameworks for mental health. She has over 150 publications and is Managing Editor of the journal *Early Intervention in Psychiatry*.

Simon Rice is a Principal Research Fellow and Associate Professor at Orygen; Centre for Youth Mental Health at the University of Melbourne. He is a practicing Clinical Psychologist with clinical expertise in management of youth mood disorders, suicide prevention, and family-based intervention for depression. Simon is a member of the International Olympic Committee (IOC) Expert Consensus Group for Elite Athlete Mental Health. He had published over 150 scientific papers related to mental health, including as lead author of the Athlete Psychological Strain Questionnaire – the IOC's recommended triage scale for assessing emerging mental health problems in elite athletes.

Mary Spillane is a Senior Clinical Psychologist based in Melbourne, Australia. She has extensive experience working in Clinical Psychology and works to enhance the well-being and mental health of elite athletes and teams. She has previously worked in both public and private mental health and has delivered evidence based interventions in both inpatient and outpatient settings. She has a keen interest in treating obsessive compulsive disorder and anxiety disorders generally and understanding how these conditions affect elite athletes. She is currently the Mental Health Lead at the Australian Institute of Sport, Wellbeing Coordinator at Cricket Victoria, and consults privately.

Marion Sulprizio is a research assistant and lecturer at the German Sport University Cologne; she is also working as an expert, coach, and consultant in applied sport psychology and has a degree in psychology (diploma) and systemic coaching. The main topics of her work are mental health, prevention of stress, and motivation in elite sport. She has the position of a Managing Director of the German initiative *MentalEmpowerment* – mental health in elite sport. In the past she was both athlete and coach in competitive handball.

Varley Teoldo da Costa, Ph.D. graduated in Physical Education from the Federal University of Minas Gerais (UFMG). He has a Master's degree in Physical Education (UFMG), Ph.D. in Sports Sciences (UFMG) with an emphasis on Soccer and Sport Psychology. He is currently Associate Professor at the School of Physical Education, Physiotherapy and Occupational Therapy (UFMG). He is a Professor in the Sports Science Program/ UFMG (master's and doctorate); Coordinator of UFMG Soccer Science Center and Sport Psychology Laboratory/ LAPES/ UFMGl; Board Member the Brazilian Association of Studies in Sports and Exercise Psychology (ABEPPEx) and Iberoamerican Society of Sports Psychology (SIPD); and Professor at the CBF Academy for football coaches licenses.

Tshepang Tshube, Ph.D. is a Senior Lecturer in the Department of Sport Science at the University of Botswana. Tshube holds a Ph.D. in Sport and Exercise Psychology from Michigan State University. He is an active researcher in Southern Africa published in areas of mental skills, dual-career, life skills, coach-athlete relations, and elite athlete retirement transition. In addition to his academic work, Tshube is a member of the Botswana National Olympic Committee High-Performance Commission. He has consulted with Team Botswana at major international games including the 2016 Olympic Games, 2018 Commonwealth Games and several Africa Championships.

Krista Van Slingerland is a Ph.D. candidate in the School of Human Kinetics at the University of Ottawa, where she also completed a Master's degree. As the co-founder and Executive Director of the Canadian Centre for Mental Health and Sport (CCMHS), Krista is contributing to both research and practice that she hopes will advance the fi eld of mental health in sport in Canada.

Fabrízio Veloso Rodrigues, Ph.D. is a psychologist and neuropsychologist, and has a Master's degree in Behavioral Sciences at the University of Brasilia (UnB), Doctor's degree in Neuroscience and Behavior at the University of Sao Paulo (USP). He began his studies in sport psychology in 1998, in the city of Brasília. He works at the Brazilian Paralympic Committee since 2017, elaborating and applying a mental training program for high-performance athletes.

Ciro Winckler is Associative Professor of S ã o Paulo Federal University (UNIFESP); Professor of the Post Graduate Program in Human Movement Sciences at the S ã o Paulo Federal University in Santos, Brazil; Member of Board at the Brazilian Paralympic Academy/ Brazilian Paralympic Committee; High Performance Manager of Brazilian Paralympic Committee, 2017–2020; Member of IPC Athletics Coaches Advisory Group, 2013–2015; Brazilian Athletics Paralympic Manager, 2004–2016 at five Paralympic Games (Sidney, Athens, Beijing, London, Rio) and Participation in Paralympic and Olympic Athletics Word Championships.

Aline Arias Wolff, Ph.D. is a clinical sport psychologist, with a Master's degree and Ph.D. in Psychology at Federal University of Rio de Janeiro (UFRJ). She has been Manager of Brazilian Olympic Committee (COB) psychology service since 2014 and is Professor of the Cognitive Behavioral Specialization program at Pontificia Universidade Católica do Rio de Janeiro (PUC-RIO); Cognitive Behavioral Therapist and Emotion Focused Therapist level II (in training) and certified experiential therapist and supervisor for TFE Brazil.

Notes

1 Lu, F., Gill, L., Yang, M., Lee, P., Hsu, Y., Chiu, Y., & Kuan, G. (2018). Measuring Athletic Mental Energy (AME): Instrument development and validation. *Frontiers in Psychology 9*, 2363. DOI:10.3389/fpsyg.2018.02363.

2 Chiu, S. S., Hsu, Y. W., Chiu, Y. H., Chou, C. C., Gill, D. L., & Lu, F. J. H. (2020). Seeking positive strengths in buffering athletes' life stress-burnout relationship: The moderating roles of athletic mental energy. *Frontiers in Psychology 10*, 1–12. doi: 10.3389/fpsyg.2019.03007.

SERIES FOREWORD

Athlete mental health is a subject area for sport psychology researchers and practitioners alike, that has been considered, directly and indirectly, for five decades. Some of the earlier discussions were focused on athlete retirement, a partial consideration of athlete career transition and athlete development. Formative authors of this topic found that high-performance athletes who retired of their own volition were more likely to experience an effective, smooth, and expedited transition to the next stage in their lives, be it continuing education, the launch into a professional career, or further post-athletic career options. The opposite pathway to an effective athlete transition is an ineffective, and to some degree, unexpected transition. When athletes fail to plan for their post-athletic career lives well in advance of transition, the pathway to the next stage in their lives proves to be tumultuous and psychologically challenging. Some of them attempt to remain athletes and to extend their athletic careers beyond their prime, and at a point in their inevitable future, are de-selected. The troubling part of career de-selection for many is that athletic identities can be sizeable as compared to broader personhood given the intensive investment of time and energy each day, sometimes over decades. Every person has multiple sites that together tell a full story of who the person is. The athlete is a person first, though some centralize the athlete condition disproportionately as their personhood.

The opening chapter of this volume titled "Setting the scene: Mental health in elite sport" reveals that the topic of athlete mental health has grown considerably since the earliest of discussions. Recently, mental health is often considered in the context of self-regulation and coping (e.g., WHO). From such a perspective it is based on one's own intentions and plans and embedded in social values and cultural conditions. The field of sport psychology has grown, and enveloped in the broader field, there is now considerable attention placed on athlete mental health, taking into account the individual conditions, social conditions, and the training and competition environment. The co-editors of this volume (i.e., opening authors) have reviewed the recent position stands about athlete mental health, written by scholars and practitioners from the Federation of European Sport Psychologists, the International Olympic Committee, domestic/national organizations, such as the Canadian Centre for Athlete Mental Health, and the founding organization of this book series, the International Society of Sport Psychology. The expanding discourse focused on athlete mental health continues to grow in leaps and bounds. Recently, Team Denmark (2018) and the United States Olympic Committee (2019) hosted successive International Society of Sport Psychology World Think Tanks, where international sport psychology societies were invited to send a participant to what has become an annual event. The resulting discussions have enriched our field in the form of two consensus statements focused on elite athlete mental health and athlete mental health within an Olympic quadrennium. The findings unequivocally point to an expansive field, though also one fertile and in need of exploration. Topic areas related to scope of practice, the athlete condition, effective social support services, stigmatization/de-stigmatization, all inclusive of nationalities, leave the sport psychology professional enthused to engage with this book.

The current compilation is edited by Carsten Hvid Larsen, Karin Moesch, Natalie Durand-Bush, and Kristoffer Henriksen, respected scholar-practitioners from three countries. The book co-editors have undertaken a unique enterprise, which we believe is much needed; they have considered mental health drawing upon a vast number of international perspectives. The current moment is one in need of our civility, where inclusiveness is a heavily discussed topic and people are re-conceptualizing their own place in the world. People across societies are attempting to find ways to be more inclusive of cultural identities, including athletes' identities. However, to be inclusive, they must first become aware and in support of our respective similarities and differences. Inclusiveness is a global necessity, and it is in keeping with the International Society of Sport Psychology's Mission since ISSP's founding, in 1965. Athlete mental health is a unique status experienced by each athlete, but to varying degrees in a given moment. A focus on mental health is necessary and overdue. We must understand what sport psychology consultants' objectives should be and where (and how) we can support each performer's excellence – by supporting human betterment in and through sport. Presently, there is not enough understanding of potential pathways of how to foster athlete mental health and, when mental health is in strain, how to support the performer in the quest for an improved human condition. The current book is a necessary addition to each sport psychology professional's and student's readings. Professionals in sport psychology have the opportunity to understand that athlete mental health is more than a mono-cultural series of strategies. There are unlocked answers to the rapidly emerging topic of athlete mental health found in the current edited book. We, as the series co-editors, are grateful to the co-editors and their authors for their novel contributions. We believe that the current contribution will impact athletes, coaches, sport psychology consultants, sport organizations, and scholars for years to come. Athlete mental health is a worldwide discourse, and the current book provides so many openings and insights that must spur international discourse and collaborations.

Robert J. Schinke, Athanasios Papioannou, and Thomas Schack
Series Co-Editors

1

SETTING THE SCENE

Mental health in elite sport

Carsten Hvid Larsen, Andreas Küttel, Karin Moesch, Natalie Durand-Bush, and Kristoffer Henriksen

Elite sport, and sports in general, offer many opportunities to promote mental health (MH). The positive effects of regular exercise on MH and well-being are well established for both youth and adults (Biddle, 2016). Moreover, the sporting context can be an excellent psychosocial-emotional training ground where players engage in teamwork and social interactions, and acquire psychological and emotional skills such as self-awareness, discipline, resilience, motivation, communication, planning, and time management, to name a few (Aquilina, 2013).

Despite the potential positive influence of sport, we have seen in recent years several examples of elite athletes experiencing MH problems, which corresponds with research findings demonstrating significant levels of mental ill-health among some athlete populations (e.g., Foskett & Longstaff, 2018; Gouttebarge, Castadelli-Maia, Gorczynski, Hainline, Hitchcock, Kerkhoffs, Rice, & Reardon, 2019). How can we best understand this? Is a downside to the intense involvement in organized sport needed for athletes to be successful? Increasingly, competitive international sport has led to intensified pressure on Olympic and professional athletes. We are witnessing increasing training loads and performance demands that inevitably present threats to athletes' MH. Just as physical training must be balanced with adequate recovery to see progress, psychological demands must also be balanced with recovery and mental performance and MH support. But which strategies are most suitable for MH promotion and prevention, and how can they be organized and implemented? What course of action should be taken when MH challenges become illnesses and what factors must be taken into consideration for the treatment of mental disorders in elite sport contexts? These are some of the key questions that motivated this book.

A comprehensive lens to address mental health

There has long existed the assumption that because elite athletes are in peak physical health, they are impervious to MH challenges (Morgan, 1979). But with emerging evidence regarding the prevalence of mental illness in athletes and the increasing number of high-profile athletes publicly talking about their mental challenges and disorders, this assumption is merely but a myth. The elite sport context consists of a unique range of stressors that may negatively influence athletes' MH (Arnold & Fletcher, 2012; Schinke et al., 2017), for example overtraining (Kenttä, Hassmen, & Raglin, 2006), injury (Putukian, 2016), coaching style (Blanchard, Amiot, Perreault, Vallerand, & Provencher, 2009; Reinboth & Duda, 2006), expectations of significant others for success (Mountjoy, Rhind, Tilvas, & Leglise, 2015), and transitions through and out of sport (Kuettel, Boyle, & Schmid, 2017; Park, Lavallee, & Tod, 2013). There are also aspects of elite sport participation that can complicate the diagnosis and treatment of athletes experiencing mental illness, such as athletic identity, competitive anxiety, eating and weight requirements, sleep and recovery, and competition and travel schedules (Bär & Markser, 2013; Glick & Horsfall, 2009).

As co-editors of this book, we support the notions that winning "at any cost" is incompatible with a modern responsible sport system that values the human behind the performer and that MH is a core component of any culture of excellence (Henriksen et al., 2019). After being involved in the context of elite sport over many years in our respective countries, it is fair to say that most clubs, national governing bodies, and Olympic committees acknowledge that MH and performance are interlinked. It is our collective view that the relative failure to address MH in sport over the years has been in part due to prevailing stigma and false misconceptions that athletes have an indestructible psyche. However, in today's society, gaps in adequate MH support are more due to a lack of knowledge, skills, and funding within organizations. Proper care for the MH and psychosocial and emotional development of athletes are generally perceived to be beneficial for all involved. They may contribute to athletes' performances, the longevity of their career, the quality of their career transitions, and better outcomes upon career termination.

Also, there appears to be increasing evidence that at both the club and national governing body level, considerable interest exists in supporting the MH of players in professional sports (Mitchell et al., 2014). However, the substantive growth in sports science provision in many clubs across Europe (Nesti & Sully, 2014) has not included a similar expansion in mental performance and MH support. Research has revealed that clubs are looking for a lead in how to address the issue of psychological support to enhance the well-being and performance of players while competing for their club and when they exit (e.g., Brown & Portrac, 2009). Yet, the answer is not that simple. Different sports, countries, and athlete populations present multiple contexts that impact how support can be implemented, and there is no one-size-fits-all solution. We envisage that this tour around the world leaves the reader with an understanding of the massive global differences in MH service provision within different contexts, and organizations. The overall aim of the book is to provide researchers, practitioners, coaches, and students with relevant knowledge, and strategies to address MH in elite sport across a variety of contexts.

"Backdrop: The ISSP Think Tank on mental health in elite sport"

During the last years, the world of sport gained increased awareness of MH. In September 2018, on the initiative of the International Society of Sport Psychology (ISSP), the first international Think Tank on Athlete Mental Health was held at the University of Southern Denmark. The purpose of the Think Tank was to unify major sport psychology organizations in a discussion of the current status and future challenges of research and applied aspects of athlete MH, and to develop recommendations for sport organizations and researchers. The Think Tank participants were selected to secure research expertise, applied experience, global representation, and collaboration between key organizations. The ISSP, the European Federation of Sport Psychology (FEPSAC), the Association of Applied Sport Psychology (AASP), and the Asian South Pacific Association of Sport Psychology (ASPASP) were asked to nominate an expert from their organization. Selected professional sport organizations and national Olympic Committees were also offered a voice in this Think Tank. After the meeting, a statement representing the consensus views of the invited group was published (Henriksen et al., 2019). In the statement, the contributors presented six propositions and recommendations to inspire researchers in their work to understand and investigate athlete MH, and sport organizations in their efforts to build elite sport environments that optimally nourish athletes' MH. These propositions are:

1. MH is a core component of a culture of excellence.
   Sporting organizations, practitioners, and researchers should pay attention to athlete MH in all their work to promote athletic performance.
2. MH in a sport context should be better defined.
   Researchers should develop a clear definition of MH in sport (1) as more than the absence of mental ill health, (2) as contextualized, (3) as decoupled from performance, and (4) in ways that create space for a variety of emotional states and for periods in which athletes are not able to contribute productively to their team's on-field performance.
3. Research on MH in sport should broaden the scope of assessment.
   Researchers should: (1) develop sport-specific measures of MH; (2) develop tools to screen both athletes and organizations for risk and protective factors; (3) employ multiple methods; (4) provide room for individual narratives that may expand our conceptualization of MH; and (5) recognize the contextual nature of MH.
4. Athlete MH is a major resource for the whole athletic career and the life afterwards.
   Sport organizations should view their athletes as whole persons and in a life-span perspective, and be extra careful to promote health and thriving, and to reduce threats to MH, during difficult career transitions. Career transition researchers are recommended to pay more direct attention to how MH may affect athletic careers and how career transitions may affect MH.
5. The environment can nourish or malnourish athlete MH.
   Researchers should investigate the features of sporting environments that nourish and malnourish athletes' MH with the aim to develop guidelines to inform sport environments, such as federations, clubs, and talent academies. Sport organizations should consider MH as a criterion of their effectiveness and use the guidelines to openly and critically review the degree to which their environment is a resource for their athletes' MH.
6. MH is everybody's business but should be overseen by one or a few specified members.
   Sport organizations should: (a) employ one or a few well-trained, licensed, or certified and experienced professionals who have the MH of the athletes as a primary focus (mental health officer, MHO), and (b) collaborate with universities to develop specific courses to ensure properly educated people are available to fulfill the role.

Building upon the work of the first ISSP Think Tank in Denmark, the international members of the second 2019 ISSP Think Tank focused on "Mental Health and the Games" using a series of directed small group discussions to address the practical challenges and opportunities facing organizations in building an effective MH support program for Olympians and Paralympians. The aim of the discussions was to develop support strategies for the unique world of Olympic and Paralympic athletes. The Think Tank resulted in a second consensus statement (Henriksen et al., 2020) and an executive summary report (McCann et al., 2020). Think Tank members stressed that The Games and MH are interrelated, because athletes committing wholeheartedly to an Olympic/Paralympic pursuit are at increased risk of high life stress (Henriksen et al., 2020). The participants divided the quadrennial into three main phases (i.e., pre-, during, and post-Games) and for each phase listed key opportunities and challenges, described how the sport environment could nourish or malnourish athlete MH, and discussed collaboration within expert support teams.

This book is a natural extension of the two Think Tanks and was initiated based on the discussions. Whereas the Consensus Statements set a clear direction and presented bold propositions, they did not provide contextualized practical examples.

An inclusive definition of mental health

According to the World Health Organization (WHO), MH is "a state of well-being in which the individual realizes his or her own abilities, can cope with the normal stresses of life, can work productively and fruitfully, and is able to make a contribution to his or her community" (WHO, 2014). Notably, a more inclusive definition was put forth by Galderisi et al. (2015) that accounts for differences in values, cultures, and social background, and curbs any restrictive and culture-bound statements. This definition is highly appropriate given the multicultural perspectives and concrete examples provided in this book to help promote MH and to prevent and treat mental disorders in sport across nations; however, it is not sport-specific:

> Mental health is a dynamic state of internal equilibrium which enables individuals to use their abilities in harmony with universal values of society. Basic cognitive and social skills; ability to recognize, express and modulate one's own emotions, as well as empathize with others; flexibility and ability to cope with adverse life events and function in social roles; and harmonious relationship between body and mind represent important components of MH which contribute, to varying degrees, to the state of internal equilibrium.

These authors deemed the expression "universal values" necessary to recognize values that have worldwide significance, such as respect and care for oneself and others, connectedness between people, respect for the environment, and respect for one's own freedom and that of others. The notion of "dynamic state of internal equilibrium" highlights the reality that certain life events and periods (e.g., adolescence, marriage, retirement) can rupture one's equilibrium and necessitate the search for a new one (e.g., new baseline). In this process, it is normal for one to experience a range of emotions such as fear, anger, sadness, and grief, and to strive to restore one's equilibrium in a timely manner through resilience. Reference to "cognitive skills" (e.g., ability to pay attention, remember and organize information, solve problems, and make decisions) and "social skills" (e.g., ability to use verbal/non-verbal abilities to communicate and interact with others) denote their importance to function well in all aspects of everyday life, and support the value of mental and social skills training – the crux of sport psychology practitioners' focus. The word "basic" conveys that a minimal degree of ability is required for functioning and that while mild impairment may be normal, moderate to severe impairment likely signifies the need for external support and incentives. "Emotional regulation" (i.e., ability to recognize, express, and modulate one's own emotions) is another key component of MH impacting one's day-to-day functioning and ability to adjust to stress. Linked to this, "empathy" (i.e., ability to experience and understand what others feel without confusion between oneself and others) is a fundamental aspect of effective communication and interaction with others. "Flexibility and ability to cope with adverse events and function in social roles" underscores the importance of resilience and relationships in the maintenance of MH. However, societal and systemic patterns of stigmatization, discrimination, and exclusion impact MH outcomes and must be taken into consideration when examining one's overall functioning. Finally, the concept of a "harmonious relationship between body and mind" is in line with the notion of internal equilibrium, the importance of both mental and physical health, and points to a holistic view of how one interacts with the world.

While this definition represents a move away from the conceptualization of MH as a state of absence of mental illness (MI), Galderisi et al. (2015) reported how some of the aforementioned aspects of MH, when significantly impaired, have been associated with mental illness (MI). In this sense, MI is characterized by substantial alterations in one's feeling, thinking, and behaving, leading to significant distress and impaired functioning in one's personal and professional activities (WHO, 2014). Although research is limited, athletes' MH has commonly been investigated through mapping symptoms of general psychological distress or the prevalence of symptoms of mental disorders (CMD; e.g., depression, anxiety, and eating disorder). As such, it can be argued that MH has often been indirectly conceptualized as the absence of such symptoms. However, assuming that all athletes who do not show or report clinical disorders are mentally healthy is too simplistic (Henriksen et al., 2019; Schinke et al., 2017). The WHO's (2014) definition of MH adopts a positive psychology perspective and represents a more holistic view of MH, emphasizing well-being as a core construct. Yet, it also raises several concerns and lends itself to potential misunderstandings when it delimits positive feelings and positive functioning as key factors for MH. For instance, in an elite sport context, it may be difficult to rationalize why athletes would subject themselves to ongoing stress, discomfort, pain, and even injuries that may limit their ability to realize their full potential and to meaningfully contribute to their community. This points to the need to consider a more nuanced view of MH in which the potential for impaired functioning (i.e., MI) is also acknowledged, such as that suggested by Galderisi and colleagues (2015). MH and MI are dynamic inter-related constructs that must both be taken into consideration when examining one's overall level of functioning (Van Slingerland et al., 2019).

From an empirical standpoint, research adopting this dual lens is scarce and mostly qualitative in nature. Keyes' (2002) two-dimensional framework (see Figure 1.1), in which MH and MI are conceptualized as two separate continua, is arguably the best one to capture athletes' complete and dynamic states throughout their career. One dimension in the model refers to the presence or absence of MH while the other dimension represents the presence or absence of MI. What is noteworthy is that athletes' level of MH and MI can fluctuate at any point in time across the four quadrants depicted in Figure 1.1. For example, throughout their career, athletes may or may not have a MI and they can concurrently have languishing (poor), moderate, or flourishing (good) MH. This means that it is possible at any point in time for athletes to (a) have a MI and be flourishing (have good MH), (b) not have a mental

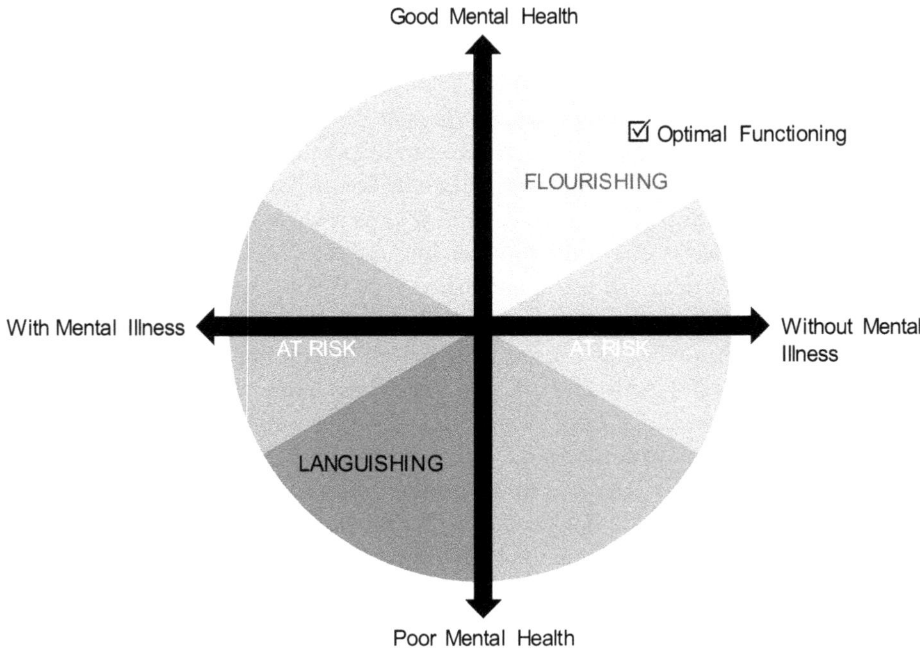

FIGURE 1.1 Keyes' (2002) two-continua model of mental health and mental illness
Source: Durand-Bush et al., 2020.

illness and be languishing (poor MH), or (c) have moderate MH, with or without a MI. Based on these different scenarios, athletes' functioning will vary and the ideal scenario is arguably the one in which they experience complete MH (i.e., flourishing, optimally functioning) without a MI.

MH is not only a reflection of the self but also the environment (e.g., culture) in which one functions. Several decades ago, Jahoda (1958) subdivided MH into the three domains of self-realization (i.e., individuals are able to fully exploit their potential), sense of mastery over the environment, and sense of autonomy (i.e., ability to identify, confront, and solve problems). However, Murphy (1978) argued that these ideas were laden with cultural values considered important by North Americans that may not be applicable in other countries and contexts. Henriksen et al. (2019) advocated for the development of a sport-specific definition of MH that transcends boundaries or may be adapted to different social values and norms. Küttel and Larsen (2019) proposed the following definition of MH in relation to elite sport, taking into consideration Keyes (2002, 2007) and the WHO's (2014) MH definitions and the high performance sport literature:

> Mental health is a dynamic state of well-being in which athletes can realize their potential, see a purpose and meaning in sport and life, experience trusting personal relationships, cope with common life stressors and the specific stressors in elite sport, and are able to act autonomously according to their values.

This definition highlights five of the six dimensions of psychological well-being put forth by Ryff (1989; autonomy, environmental mastery, personal growth, positive relations with others, purpose in life). While self-acceptance is not addressed, the definition does present MH as a dynamic state that is contingent upon staying true to one's values (e.g., personal and cultural), which is similar to what Galderisi et al. (2015) proposed. It also distinguishes that sport-specific factors must be considered when examining athletes' MH. This first sport-focused conceptualization of MH is important; however, there is value in complementing it with that of Galderisi and colleagues, to have an inclusive and comprehensive view of MH that acknowledges the potential for impaired functioning.

State of the art: Increased awareness and focus on MH in elite sport

Athletes' MH has recently attracted the attention of scholars all over the world, who have produced scientific articles and reviews, as well as position stands and consensus statements. To illustrate, when searching the Scopus Database with the search terms *("mental health") AND (athlet* OR player OR sport)* by year, Walton et al. (2020) identified 50 articles published in 2006, 150 in 2012, and nearly 400 in 2018. Looking at review papers on MH that emerged a decade ago, it can be observed that the discourse of MH in elite athletes originated from a rather limited conceptualization of athletes' MH (e.g., Bär & Markser, 2013; Glick et al., 2012; Reardon & Factor, 2010). These early reviews primarily focused on the diagnosis and medical treatment of MI (i.e., mood, anxiety, eating, addictive disorders) of athletes and concluded that more knowledge is needed about the prevalence, risk factors, and the unique experiences that athletes face concerning their MI.

In 2016, Rice et al. conducted a systematic review including 60 quantitative studies. These studies were grouped according to major MH constructs such as anger/aggression, eating disorder and body image, stress and coping, sleep, help-seeking, substance abuse, and well-being. Rice and colleagues found that the evidence base regarding the MH (i.e., well-being) of elite athletes was limited by a paucity of high-quality, systematic studies, including intervention trials. Despite these shortcomings, the authors concluded that elite athletes in general seem to experience MH issues at approximately the same level as the general population. In their meta-analysis, Gorczynski, Coyle, and Gibson (2017) further corroborated these findings by comparing mild or more severe depression between high-performance and non-athletes. Depressive symptomatology ranged from 3.7% to 26.7% for male athletes and from 9.8% to 36.5% for female athletes. Certain athletes seem to be more at-risk for specific MH disorders. For example, female athletes participating in aesthetic or leanness sports report a higher prevalence of eating disorders than other athletes and individuals in the general population (Byrne & McLean, 2002; Schaal et al., 2011; Thiemann, Legenbauer, Vocks, 2015; Kussman & Nattiv, 2016). Another systematic review on the determinants of anxiety in elite athletes was conducted by Rice and colleagues in 2019. Their narrative review of 61 studies and the meta-analyses of 27 studies indicated several general factors as being salient to symptomatic anxiety in elite athletes, including female gender, younger age, and recent experience of adverse life events. Career dissatisfaction, injuries, and athletic retirement were further determinants of anxiety among athletes. As anxiety disorders account for a large proportion of the burden of disease among all MH problems, Rice and colleagues advocated for greater attention and action to determine their prevalence and impacts on elite athlete populations. Looking beyond the disorders that got most attention in the elite sport context, a number of disorders such as ADHD and bipolar disorder have been overlooked in research in elite athletes (e.g., Lebrun & Collins, 2017; Reardon & Factor, 2010).

Küttel and Larsen (2019) conducted a scoping review on risk and protective factors for elite athletes' MH and included both quantitative and qualitative articles published from 1998 to 2018. Their review showed that the majority of the 43 studies included were of quantitative nature using a cross-sectional design with self-administered scales (e.g., Patient Health Questionnaire-9, General Anxiety Disorder-7, Center for Epistemological Study Depression Scale) to investigate the prevalence of symptoms in athletes (e.g., depression, anxiety, eating disorder) in relation to, for example, injury, critical life events, specific stressors, gender, and social support. Küttel and Larsen also highlighted that the majority (66%) of the athletes were male, and data were collected mostly in Western countries (i.e., Europe, Australia, North America). Additionally, even though only studies that labeled their sample as high-performance, elite, or professional athletes were included, the heterogeneity of the sample (both within and across studies) was rather large, which is a common problem in sport research (Swann et al., 2015). In total, across the studies, 82 correlates for MH were identified and consequently grouped into personal and environmental protective and risk factors. *Protective factors* such as autonomy, positive social relationships, and personal behavior (e.g., accepting multiple roles, setting meaningful and realistic goals) were mostly identified through qualitative studies, whereas *risk factors* (e.g., injury/concussion, overtraining, adverse life events, negative coping strategies, pressure to perform, deselection, maladaptive personality traits and identity, and stigma toward help-seeking) predominantly emerged from studies using a quantitative research design. Since only three out of the 43 studies investigated the potential influence of the sporting environment on athletes' MH, the authors emphasized that an increased focus should be placed on the environment in which the athlete develops, because a trusting and mastery-oriented climate, as opposed to a culture of "winning at all costs," has been shown to be beneficial for the MH of athletes (Ivarsson et al. 2015; Swann et al., 2018).

Another review paper discussed the role of sport coaches in promoting MH (Bissett, Kroshus, & Hebard, 2020) and highlighted that coaching education programs should not only address signs, symptoms, and referral procedures, but also provide examples of behaviors in which coaches may engage to foster a positive team culture surrounding MH. In a similar vein, Castaldelli-Maia et al. (2019) addressed the importance of coaches in their systematic review of cultural influencers and barriers to athletes seeking treatment. They indicated that coaches are in frequent contact with athletes, and thus can support and encourage acknowledgement and treatment of MH symptoms and disorders by creating a destigmatizing environment wherein MH treatment-seeking is a core function of training and self-care.

Recent consensus statements on athlete MH from international organizations, associations, and committees

Since 2017, consensus statements from different international organizations have been published regarding athletes and their MH. The ISSP presented a position stand (Schinke et al., 2017) discussing athletes' MH in relation to athletic performance, overtraining, injury, career development, culture, and identity. Emphasizing that MH should be seen as a major resource for a sustainable athletic career, Schinke and colleagues also questioned conceptualizations of MH as the absence of MI. Instead, MH should be understood on a continuum from (a) active MI, to (b) sub-syndrome illness (frequent symptoms), to (c) normal functioning (occasional symptoms), to (d) good MH (asymptomatic), and to (e) peak performance (flow or zone states). The position stand focused mostly on subclinical MH issues of athletes and ended with ten postulates aiming to inspire sport psychology researchers and practitioners to increase their contribution to athletes' long-lasting, successful, and healthy careers in sport and life.

In the position statement of the European Federation of Sport Psychology (FEPSAC), Moesch et al. (2018) provided an overview of service provision for athletes' suffering from MI (mental illness) in six European countries. They showed that competencies, certification issues, and professional boundaries of relevant service providers differ considerably across European countries. With the aim to inspire stakeholders to optimize their MH support systems, the authors suggested recommendation around education and help-seeking behavior, sport-specificity in detection and treatment of athlete MHD, and clarity of pathways and signposting by institutions and stakeholders.

In the North American context, Slingerland and colleagues (2018) postulated the following six principles of MH in high-performance sport in association with the Canadian Centre for Mental Health and Sport (CCMHS): (1) Athletes are susceptible to experiencing MH challenges and disorders; (2) Sport organizations have a duty to protect the MH of athletes; (3) Coaches have a duty to foster the MH of their athletes; (4) Competitive and high-performance athletes seeking care for MH challenges or disorders are best served by a specialized interdisciplinary MH care team; (5) Truly comprehensive integrated support teams in sport include at least one practitioner who can address MH challenges and mental illness in athletes; and (6) Institutions offering programs to train MH professionals have a duty to provide opportunities to develop sport-specific competencies. By laying a foundation for a unified discourse, these authors presented solutions to current challenges and urged the Canadian sport community to more actively challenge the status quo and move from MH *talk* to MH *action*.

The American Medical Society for Sports Medicine (AMSSM) convened a panel of experts to provide an evidence-based, best-practices document to assist sport medicine physicians and other members of the athletic care network with the detection, treatment, and prevention of MH issues in competitive athletes (Chang et al., 2019). From a medical perspective, the AMSSM advocates the important component of pharmacological treatment options including those that may be the most effective with the fewest side effects.

Acknowledging the necessity for evidence-based recommendations of a more policy-related approach to MH and awareness programs in sport, Breslin et al. (2019) published an international consensus statement intending to (a) inform those developing psychosocial or policy-related MH awareness programs, and (b) provide direction for researchers, policymakers, and practitioners working in this emerging area. The six recommendations are related to (1) the definition of MH awareness; (2) standards for data collection, analysis and reporting; (3) the appropriate selection of theoretical models and theories; (4) the minimal competencies of professionals involved in sport to support MH in sport; (5) acknowledging diversity (age, gender, culture) when providing guidance; and (6) identifying the role of parents, officials, coaches, and athletes in the cocreation of MH promotion in various sport settings.

In 2018, The International Olympic Committee (IOC) invited a range of worldwide experts (psychiatrists, psychologists, sport medicine physicians, exercise scientists) to conduct a systematic review on 20 selected topics related to specific MH symptoms and disorders in elite athletes (e.g., sleep disorder, post-traumatic stress disorder, bipolar and psychotic disorders, substance use, anxiety, depression, and sleep disorder; Reardon et al., 2019). Aside from these issues, the authors discussed major stressors and key environmental factors that influence elite athlete MH such as discrimination, harassment and abuse. These can potentially impact physical (e.g., illness and injuries), cognitive (e.g., low self-esteem), emotional (e.g., volatile mood states), behavioral (e.g., drop-out), and social (e.g., social exclusion) dimensions of athlete MH and lead to MI (e.g., anxiety, depression). The IOC consensus statement concluded that MH is an integral dimension of elite athlete well-being and performance and cannot be separated from physical health. Therefore, MH assessment and management in elite athletes should be as commonplace and accessible as their other medical care and elite athletes ideally should have access to the best interdisciplinary care teams.

General and sport-specific assessment of MH and MI in elite athletes

Attempting to measure psychosocial phenomena such as MH is a complex and difficult endeavor, particularly in a specialized context like high-performance sport. A relevant question and proposition put forth in most of the above-mentioned consensus statements pertains to the definition and underlying dimensions of MH. Related to this are different ways to measure both MH and MI in the context of elite sport. To be able to develop optimal assessment methodologies and screening tools, a better understanding of the unique symptom manifestations in athletes is needed, which may require both qualitative and quantitative study across countries and cultures (Reardon et al., 2019).

Interestingly, some evidence suggests that athletes may be unmotivated to complete general scales due to perceived stigma and they may not be forthright in their responses to these instruments because there is no direct connection between the assessment of MH and sport performance (Donohue et al., 2018). Therefore, the development of sport-specific measures of MH must be prioritized to advance knowledge and have the capacity to more effectively support athletes' health and performance. Giles et al. (2019) provided an overview of eight different scales (i.e., Mental Health Continuum Short-Form (MHC-SF); Warwick-Edinburg Mental Well-being Scale; Flourishing Scale) used to measure MH/well-being, however, these are not specific to sport. Recognizing this, the authors highlighted four key areas of concern relevant for measuring well-being in elite athletes: (1) conceptual and theoretical issues (e.g., to encompass a combination of both hedonic and eudaimonic components); (2) item development issues (e.g., contextual phrasing of items, items related to both global and contextual levels of well-being); (3) measurement and scoring issues (e.g., bias in retrospective questionnaires, scale polarity, and length); and (4) analytical and statistical issues (e.g., factor structure, reliability, trade-off between shorter and more practical measures on the one hand, and longer and typically more reliable scales on the other). Giles and colleagues challenged researchers to consider whether the highest levels of well-being are always desirable and realistic, particularly given the potentially complex relationship between athletic performance and MH at the highest level. This raises ethical questions that require serious debate, as it suggests that athletes should be ready to sacrifice their MH to achieve the highest levels in sport.

In line with Keyes' (2002) dual-continua model, there is a need for sound assessments for not only MH but also MI in sport. Screening for MH is an important prevention strategy, as early identification and treatment can reduce the severity and duration of symptomatology. Some instruments were developed by researchers to measure MH challenges in sport performers, mainly in the US collegiate athletic context. For example, Donohue and colleagues (2007, 2018) put forth an empirical screening method to guide MH referrals in collegiate athletes. The Sport Interference Checklist (SIC; Donohue et al., 2007) contains 26 items that ask how often certain situations/thoughts (e.g., "over concerned or worry too much about what others think about my performance," "being homesick or lacking close social supports") interfere with athletes' performance during training or competition, and if athletes would seek professional help for this if possible. The value of this checklist is its focus on sport and performance-related factors, although it does not directly target sub-clinical or clinical symptoms. Another screening tool for athlete MH was developed and validated by Rice, Parker, and colleagues (2019). The Athletes Psychological Strain Questionnaire (APSQ) contains ten items resulting in a three-factor solution, with subscales assessing self-regulation, performance, and external coping. The APSQ showed both high sensitivity (i.e., hit rate) and high specificity (i.e., correct rejection rate) relative to those experiencing elevated distress, as identified by a general distress scale. Hence, in combination with other tools, this measure could assist in early identification and provision of support to improve the MH of athletes, even though it does not measure symptoms related to MH challenges per se.

Concerning MI-related measures, a ten-item self-report depression screening tool (e.g., "I rarely get pleasure from competing anymore and have lost interest in my sport") was developed by Baron et al. (2013) for the athletic population, which can be used prior to evaluation by MH professionals. Burnout is a recognized MI in some countries and a widely known risk factor in elite sport (Gustafsson et al., 2011). Symptoms of burnout can be assessed using the Athlete Burnout Questionnaire (ABQ; Raedeke & Smith, 2001), a 14-item scale measuring the frequency with which athletes feel various emotions toward sport (e.g., being overly tired from sport, not performing in sport). The ABQ is comprised of three subscales: physical/emotional exhaustion, reduced accomplishment, and sport devaluation. A mean score of 3.0 or higher on physical/emotional exhaustion and reduced accomplishment scales (Cresswell & Eklund, 2006; Dubuc-Charbonneau & Durand-Bush, 2014) is typically used as a threshold to identify athletes warranting further investigation. The scale has been validated in college athletes aged 17–23 years (Raedeke & Smith, 2001).

Sleep disturbances are often reported by high-performance sport athletes. As such, it is important to have adequate measures to track this in athletes. Using the Pittsburgh Sleep Quality Index Questionnaire (Buysse, Reynolds, et al., 1989), Van Slingerland and colleagues (2019) indicated that 87% of a sample of 31 high-performance athletes seeking MH support through the CCMHS scored positive on this measure. Samuels, James, Lawson, and Meeuwisse (2016) recently put forth the Athlete Sleep Screening Questionnaire (ASSQ), which contains 16 items pertaining to respondents' sleep habits during the recent past. A sleep difficulty score is derived, which categorizes respondents as having mild, moderate, severe, or no sleep difficulties. Some items are used to assist clinicians in designing interventions and sleep optimization strategies. The ASSQ was developed for elite athletes and clinically validated with a sample of Canadian national team athletes ($N = 199$), yielding a diagnostic sensitivity of 81%, a specificity of 93%, a positive predictive value of 87%, and a negative predictive value of 90% (Bender, Lawson, Werthner, & Samuels, 2018).

A comprehensive screening program for athletes was introduced by Tomalski et al. (2019), which consists of sport psychology, sport medicine, the university counseling center and members of the athletic department's sport management team engaging in biweekly meetings to (1) identify student-athletes who are struggling in any domain (physical, psychological, academic, athletic, and/or nutritional), and (2) mobilize staff and resources, including making referrals, to provide the assistance needed by each identified student-athlete. Tomalski and colleagues proposed an 18-item instrument divided into four sections to get a comprehensive view of athletes' functioning (i.e., mind, body, performance, current health status). They

TABLE 1.1 Examples of general MI screening tools

Mental Illness Symptoms	*Screening Measure*
Attention Deficit Hyperactivity Disorder	Adult ADHD Self-Report (ASRS-6; Kessler et al., 2005)
Alcohol Use Disorder	Alcohol Use Disorder Identification Test (AUDIT-C; Bush et al., 1998)
Generalized Anxiety Disorder	Generalized Anxiety Disorder scale (GAD-7; Spitzer, Kroenke, Williams, & Lowe, 2006)
Depression	Patient Health Questionnaire (PHQ-9; Spitzer, Kroenke, & Williams, 1999)
Eating Disorder	Eating Attitudes Test (EAT-26; Garner, Olmsted, Bohr, & Garfinkel, 1982)
Obsessive-Compulsive Disorder	Florida Obsessive Compulsive Inventory (FOCI; Storch et al., 2007)
Post-Traumatic Stress Disorder	PTSD checklist (PCL-5; Blevins et al., 2015)
Sleep Disorder	Pittsburgh Sleep Quality Index Questionnaire (PSQ; Buysse, Reynolds, et al., 1989)
Substance Use Disorder	Drug Abuse Screening Test (DAST-10; Skinner, 1989)
Suicidality	Columbia-Suicide Severity Rating Scale (C-SSRS; Posner et al., 2008)

discussed different follow-up procedures after screening (e.g., face-to-face meetings with a health professional). Even though frequent screening and continually monitoring athletes' MH is important and can help to provide relevant, timely, and effective service, it demands extensive resources and staff that many institutions/clubs/academies do not have, hence making it difficult to replicate this program in other settings (Rancourt et al., 2019).

Overall, sport-specific assessment tools related to MH and MI in elite athletes remain scarce. While some progress has been made, most tools have not been widely used and tested in the sport context yet. As such, results gleaned from the use of these measures should be interpreted with caution. On the other hand, it is important to note that traditional screening tools (see examples in Table 1.1) that are extensively used and validated with the general population to detect sub-clinical and clinical symptoms of MI also bear limitations when used in elite sport contexts. For example, complex and abnormal eating patterns are common in many high-performance sports (Reardon et al., 2019). As such, athletes may obtain 'false positive' screening scores on a general tool like the Eating Attitudes Test (EAT-26; Garner, Olmsted, Bohr, & Garfinkel, 1982). Consequently, it is important to completement any data gleaned from general screening tools with a comprehensive intake interview in order to provide an accurate and holistic view of athletes' functioning.

Promotion of MH in elite athletes

Promoting the MH of athletes is a challenging endeavor, and several questions must be answered in the search for optimal ways to do so. These questions include but are not limited to: How do we reduce stigma and increase help seeking? How do we increase MH literacy in sport environments and increase the likelihood that struggling athletes will get adequate support? Who can aid in this endeavor (mental performance consultants, clinical psychologists, medical doctors, and others) and how do we make sure all efforts are properly integrated? How do we design organizational structures for monitoring, referral, and treatment? How do we create psychologically healthy and safe competitive sport environments?

There is a growing consensus that athletes struggle with MH challenges and MI at a comparable rate or slightly elevated rate than the general population (Reardon et al., 2019). Despite this identified risk, athletes tend to seek help at a lower rate than their non-athlete peers (Rice et al., 2016). Aside from the stigma associated with help-seeking in the elite sports context (Souter et al., 2018), a lack of MH services designed specifically to serve sport populations could be a contributing factor. A strategy suggested in several consensus statements and position stands (e.g., Henriksen et al., 2019; Moesch et al., 2018; Reardon et al., 2019; Schinke et al., 2017; Van Slingerland et al., 2019) aimed at preventing and treating MH symptoms and disorders in elite athletes is to employ education interventions, specifically those based on increasing MH literacy. MH literacy is defined as the "knowledge and beliefs about mental disorders which aid their recognition, management or prevention" (Jorm et al., 1997, p. 182). As Gorczynski et al. (2020) recognized, the question remains about how MH literacy in elite sport can address the unique needs of individual athletes, but also factors in their culture and environment that can impact MH symptoms and disorders. Gorczynski and colleagues emphasize that MH literacy interventions should be based on detailed knowledge of developmental, cultural, and social issues related to sport participation and systemic issues within sport settings and organizations. Furthermore, these interventions should be designed in a manner that takes due account of organizational goals, whereby organizations learn to identify and address MH symptoms and create sport environments in which individuals can thrive.

Along these lines, Purcell et al. (2019) advocated for an early intervention framework to increase awareness for elite athletes' MH aiming at (a) helping athletes develop a range of self-management skills that they can utilize to manage psychological distress, (b) equipping key stakeholders in the elite sporting environment to better recognize and respond to concerns regarding athletes' MH, and (c) highlighting the need for specialized multi- and inter-disciplinary teams or skilled MH professionals to manage athletes with severe or complex mental disorders. The triangle-shaped framework has the *preventative or foundational components* at its base, consisting of MH literacy building, individual athlete development and skill acquisition, and MH screening and feedback. The next level is termed *indicated (at-risk) prevention components*, which comprise early detection and identification by coaches, sports medicine staff, or physiotherapists. The third level is named *early intervention* for emerging or existing MH problems, where typically structured clinical interventions for mild to moderate symptoms are addressed. The fourth and top level of the framework refer to the *specialized MH care* required for athletes with severe or complex psychopathology. The IOC Expert Consensus Statement provides a summary of recommended clinical interventions for a range of mental disorders, including bipolar, psychotic, eating and depressive disorders, and suicidality (Reardon et al., 2019).

In addition to these more general recommendations and frameworks on how to promote MH (literacy) in athletes and their support staff, several specific (Routledge) books pertaining to athlete MH have been published. Edited by Breslin and Leavey (2019), the book entitled "Mental health and well-being interventions in sport" provides insight into selected case studies with different athletic populations (e.g., junior swimmers, student-athletes), programs (e.g., state of mind program), and interventions (e.g., rational emotive behavioral therapy). The book "Psychological health and well-being in high-level athletes" by Nick Gall (2020) provides further case examples of athletes dealing with performance pressure, injury, abuse, and critical career transitions, as well as helpful guidelines on how to work with athletes in such situations and circumstances. In their book *Mindfulness and Acceptance in Sport*, which is grounded in acceptance-based cognitive behavioral approaches, Henriksen, Hansen, and Larsen (2019) describe several interventions and cases concerning athletes' performance and MH. The book presents practical examples and models designed to clarify values, defuse from unhelpful thoughts, accept difficult emotions, and use mindfulness exercises to hone the skill of present-moment focus. These interventions can potentially improve athletic performance *and* thriving for athletes who are exposed to omnipresent stressors in elite sports.

A reader's guide

The present book is part of the ISSP book series. The ISSP is a worldwide organization of scholars and practitioners explicitly concerned with sport psychology and devoted to promoting research, practice, and development in the discipline of sport psychology throughout the world. The international perspective and recognition that sport psychology is always culturally situated and must be contextually appropriate is a foundation for the ISSP and for this book. We believe the book will also be of inspiration for people working in other performance domains such as music, medicine, the performing arts, and business.

By providing a focused state of the art overview of MH research, models, and approaches in elite sport, the present introductory chapter sets the scene for the book. Beyond this opening, the book is divided into two main parts.

Part I globally focuses on MH service provision structures and cases specific to several world regions and countries. The Chapters make reference to the terminology presented in Chapter 1 and illustrate how opportunities and challenges of each national structure and program are contingent upon context and culture.

Part I comprises six chapters. In Chapter 2, Marion Sulprizio and colleagues describe two German initiatives, *mentaltalent* and *MentalEmpowerment*, which aim to systematically structure and provide sport psychological coaching in order to promote MH from a scientific perspective. In Chapter 3, Tshepang Tshube and colleagues present an illustrative and fascinating glimpse into the MH issues of elite athletes in sub-Saharan Africa, and discuss how socio-cultural and spiritual issues in sub-Saharan sports have immense impact on successful interventions in that region. Franco Noce and colleagues, in Chapter 4, provide an overview of how elite sport is organized in Brazil and how the major Brazilian sport organizations approach the MH domain. They further address practitioners' challenges and opportunities in their profession. Göran Kenttä and Karin Hyland describe in Chapter 5 the Swedish model of MI and their experiences of establishing a clinic for coaches and athletes. In Chapter 6, Lisa Olive and colleagues call for models of MH care that can identify and respond to MH needs. They illustrate how the Australian Institute of Sport (AIS) developed and implemented the MH Referral Network they proposed. Next, in Chapter 7, Natalie Durand-Bush and Krista Van Slingerland provide an overview of pathways for MH service provision in Canada. They share the contributions of the Canadian Centre for Mental Health and Sport (CCMHS), a specialized national hub providing MH services to competitive and high-performance athletes and coaches. This tour around the world leaves the reader with an understanding of the massive global differences in MH service provision.

Part II focuses on specific MH interventions across countries. The chapters similarly use the terminology introduced in Chapter 1, but also illustrate specific case studies and interventions as influenced by the local context and culture. Part II is comprised of four chapters. In Chapter 8, Alexander Cohen describes a case study in which he applied Acceptance and Commitment Therapy (ACT) for health anxiety and performance. This case illustrates the versatility of ACT in addressing complex health anxiety issues while simultaneously facilitating greater performance readiness in training and competition. Drawing on the Asian culture, Frank J. H. Lu describes in Chapter 9 how coaches' attitudes and behaviors influence athlete's MH in the unique context of Taiwanese elite sport. Touching upon the development of a collaborative care system, Samuel Cumming and colleagues in Chapter 10 present a case study to illustrate the MH support available to athletes within the High Performance System (HPS) in the UK. Additionally, they demonstrate a recommended approach to supporting athletes who experience crisis whilst traveling abroad. In the final chapter (Chapter 11), we draw conclusions from the chapters of the book and provide perspectives for future research and applied practice of MH in elite sport.

Epilogue: Moving the field forward

We already know a lot about MH in elite sport, but there is likely even more that we do not know and numerous perplexing dilemmas still exist. We believe the present book has the potential to move the field yet another notch forward.

We know that elite athletes are not immune to suffering from MH issues. In fact, we know that prevalence corresponds quite well to those of the general population. Unfortunately, much of the research relies on instruments that are not designed for sport and perhaps do not reflect the nature of elite sport very well. Although the present book does not necessarily introduce new scientific tools or procedures, we believe the diversity and complexity of the knowledge, and examples provided in each chapter of the book will lead to a deeper understanding of the opportunities, limitations, and challenges involved in investigating and providing a comprehensive view of MH in elite athlete populations.

We know that many current definitions of MH are ill-aligned with the nature of elite sport. What may be seen as a problematic symptom in daily life may be seen as an accepted part of life in elite sport and vary hugely depending on the time of season (off-season vs. peak competitive season). We believe that the ideas and cases brought forth in this book might help readers gain a better understanding of how MH can really be understood in the competitive world of sport.

We know that MH is deeply contextualized and how it is fostered will vary depending on contexts. Individual (e.g., race, gender), environmental (e.g., national, political, sport-specific), and developmental (e.g., age, career phase) factors all shape athletes' lived experience of MH. We believe that by providing a host of accounts and examples, the book will add to our understanding of the contextualized nature of MH.

Finally, we know that although MH is the business of everybody in the sport context, it must be professionally overseen. Organizations have a responsibility to create an elite sport environment that supports athlete MH, and all have role to play (e.g., coaches, MH practitioners, medical staff, managers, dual career support providers). Organizations have a responsibility to provide the structures and resources to promote early identification and effective treatment of athletes at risk, cultivate help-seeking, and build MH literacy. We recognize, however, that the systems set in place to support athlete MH worldwide must vary to account for cultural and organizational differences. Therefore, this book does not give *the answer* to how we should organize prevention and treatment of MH issues in elite athlete populations. We believe, however, that the excellent examples from different sports and countries shared throughout this book will inspire practitioners and researchers to search for their own context-specific relevant answers.

Enjoy your read.

Glossary

AASP	The Association of Applied Sport Psychology
AMSSM	The American Medical Society for Sports Medicine
APSQ	The Athletes Psychological Strain Questionnaire
ASPASP	The Asian South Pacific Association of Sport Psychology
CCMHS	Canadian Centre for Mental Health and Sport
CMD	Common mental disorder
FEPSAC	The European Federation of Sport Psychology
IOC	The International Olympic Committee
ISSP	The International Society of Sport Psychology
MH	Mental health
MI	Mental illness
MHC-SF	Mental Health Continuum Short-Form
SIC	The Sport Interference Checklist
WHO	World Health Organization

References

Aquilina, D. (2013). A study of the relationship between elite athletes' educational development and sporting performance, *International Journal of History in Sport 30*, 374–392.

Arnold, R., & Fletcher, D. (2012). A research synthesis and taxonomic classification of the organizational stressors encountered by sport performers. *Journal of Sport and Exercise Psychology 34*(3), 397–429. Doi: 10.1123/jsep.34.3.397.

Bär, K.-J., & Markser, V. Z. (2013). Sport specificity of mental disorders: The issue of sport psychiatry. *European Archives of Psychiatry and Clinical Neuroscience 263*, 205–210.

Baron, D. A., Baron, S. H., Tompkins, J., & Polat, A. (2013). Assessing and treating depression in athletes. In D. A. Baron, C. L. Reardon, & S. H. Baron (Eds.), *Clinical sports psychiatry: An international perspective* (pp. 65–78). West Sussex: Wiley.

Bender, A. M., Lawson, D., Werthner, P., & Samuels, C. H. (2018). The clinical validation of the Athlete Sleep Screening Questionnaire: An instrument to identify athletes that need further sleep assessment. *Sports Medicine – Open, 4*. doi:10.116/s40798-018-0140-5.

Biddle, S. (2016). Physical activity and mental health: Evidence growing. *World Psychiatry, 15*, 176–177. Doi: 10.1002/wps.20331.

Bissett, J. E., Kroshus, E., & Hebard, S. (2020). Determining the role of sport coaches in promoting athlete mental health: A narrative review and Delphi approach. *BMJ Open Sport & Exercise Medicine, 6*.

Blanchard, C. M., Amiot, C. E., Perreault, S., Vallerand, R. J., & Provencher, P. (2009). Cohesiveness, coach's interpersonal style and psychological needs: Their effects on self-determination and athletes' subjective well-being. *Psychology of Sport and Exercise 10*, 545–551. https://doi.org/10.1016/j.psychsport.2009.02.005.

Blevins, C. A., Weathers, F. W., Davis, M. T., Witte, T. K., & Domino, J. L. (2015). The posttraumatic stress disorder checklist for DSM-5 (PCL-5): Development and initial psychometric evaluation. *Journal of Traumatic Stress, 28*, 489–498. doi: 10.1002/jts.22059.

Breslin, G., & Leavey, G. (2019). *Mental health and well-being interventions in sport: Research, theory and practice*. London: Routledge.

Breslin, G., Shannon, S., Haughey, T., Sarju, N., Neill, D., Leavey, G., & Lawlor, M. (2019). Athlete and non-athlete student intentions to self-manage mental health: Applying the integrated behaviour change model to the state of mind programme. *Journal of Applied Sport Psychology 33*(1), 1–36.

Brown, G., & Potrac, P. (2009). 'You've not made the grade, son': De-selection and identity disruption in elite level youth football. *Soccer & Society 10*, 143–159.

Bush, K., Kivlahan, D. R., McDonell, M. B., McDonnell, M. B., Fihn, S. D., & Bradley, K. A. (1998). The AUDIT alcohol consumption questions (AUDIT-C): An effective brief screening test for problem drinking. *Archives of Internal Medicine 3*, 1789–1795. doi: 10.1001/archinte.158.16.1789.

Buysse, D. J., Reynolds, C. F., Monk, T. H., Berman, S. R., Kupfer, D. J. (1989). The Pittsburgh sleep quality index: A new instrument for psychiatric practice and research. *Psychiatry Research 28*, 193–213. doi: 10.1016/0165-1781(89)90047-4.

Byrne, S., & McLean, N. (2002). Elite athletes: Effects of the pressure to be thin. *Journal of Science and Medicine in Sport 5*, 80–94. doi: 10.1016/s1440-2440(02)80029-9.

Castaldelli-Maia, J. M., e Gallinaro, J. G. de M., Falcão, R. S., Gouttebarge, V., Hitchcock, M. E., Hainline, B., … Stull, T. (2019). Mental health symptoms and disorders in elite athletes: A systematic review on cultural influencers and barriers to athletes seeking treatment. *British Journal of Sports Medicine 53*, 707–721.

Chang, C., Putukian, M., Aerni, G., Diamond, A., Hong, G., Ingram, Y., Reardon, C. L., & Wolanin, A. (2019). Mental health issues and psychological factors in athletes: Detection, management, effect on performance and prevention: American Medical Society for Sports Medicine Position Statement-Executive Summary. *British Journal of Sports Medicine 54*, 216–220. doi: 10.1136/bjsports-2019-.

Cresswell, S. L., & Eklund, R. C. (2006). The nature of player burnout in rugby: Key characteristics and attributions. *Journal of Applied Sport Psychology 18*, 219–239.

Donohue, B., Galante, M., Maietta, J., Lee, B., Paul, N., Perry, J. E., Corey, A., & Allen, D. N. (2007). Empirical development of a screening method to assist mental health referrals in collegiate athletes. *Journal of Clinical Sport Psychology 13*, 561–579. doi: https://doi.org/10.1123/jcsp.2018-0070.

Donohue, B., Gavrilova, Y., Galante, M., Gavrilova, E., Loughran, T., Scott, J., et al. (2018). Controlled evaluation of an optimization approach to mental health and sport performance. *Journal of Clinical Sport Psychology 12*(2), 121–142.

Dubuc-Charbonneau, N., Durand-Bush, N., & Forneris, T. (2014). Student-athlete burnout: Exploring levels and trends at two Canadian universities. *Canadian Journal of Higher Education 44*, 135–151.

Durand-Bush, N., & Van Slingerland, K. (2020, June). How sport leaders and coaches can preserve wealth through mental health. Invited presentation given at the Coaching Association of Canada's annual Partners Congress, Ottawa, ON, Canada.

Foskett, R., & Longstaff, F. (2018). The mental health of elite athletes in the United Kingdom. *Journal of Science and Medicine in Sport 21*, 765–770.

Galderisi, S., Heinz, A., Kastrup, M., Beezhold, J., & Sartorius, N. (2015). Toward a new definition of mental health. *World Psychiatry 14*, 231–233. doi: 10.1002/wps.20231.

Gall, N. (2020). *Psychological health and well-being in high-level athletes*. New York, NY: Routledge.

Garner, D. M., Olmsted, M. P., Bohr, Y., & Garfinkel, P. E. (1982). The eating attitudes Test: Psychometric features and clinical correlates. *Psychological Medicine 12*, 871–878. http://dx.doi.org/10.1017/S0033291700049163.

Giles, S., Fletcher, D., Arnold, R., Ashfield, A., & Harrison, J. (2019). Measuring well-being in sport performers: Where are we now and how do we progress? *Sports Medicine*. doi. https://doi.org/10.1007/s40279-020-01274-z.

Glick, I. D., & Horsfall, J. L. (2009). Psychiatric conditions in sports: Diagnosis, treatment, and quality of life. *The Physician and Sports Medicine 37*, 29–34. doi: 10.3810/psm.2001.08.913.

Glick, I. D., Stillman, M. A., Reardon, C. L., & Ritvo, E. C. (2012). Managing psychiatric issues in elite athletes. *The Journal of Clinical Psychiatry 73*, 640–644.

Gorczynski, P. F., Coyle, M., & Gibson, K. (2017). Depressive symptoms in high-performance athletes and non-athletes: A comparative meta-analysis. *British Journal of Sports Medicine 51*, 1348–1354.

Gorczynski, P., Currie, A., Gibson, K., Gouttebarge, V., Hainline, B., Castaldelli-Maia, J. M., Mountjoy, M., Purcell, R., Reardon, C. L., Rice, S., & Swartz, L. (2020). Developing mental health literacy and cultural competence in elite sport. *Journal of Applied Sport Psychology*. https://doi.org/10.1080/10413200.2020.1720045.

Gouttebarge, V., Castadelli-Maia, J. M., Gorczynski, P., Hainline, B., Hitchcock, M. E., Kerkhoffs, G. M., Rice, S. M., Reardon, C. L. (2019). Occurrence of mental health symptoms and disorders in current and former elite athletes: A systematic review and meta-analysis. *British Journal of Sports Medicine 53*, 700–707. doi:10.1136/bjsports-2019–100671.

Gustafsson, H., Kenttä, G., & Hassmén, P. (2011). Athlete burnout: An integrated model and future research directions. *International Review of Sport and Exercise Psychology 4*, 3–24. doi: https://doi.org/10.1080/1750984X.2010.541927.

Henriksen, K., Hansen, J., & Larsen, C. H. (2019). *Mindfulness and acceptance in sport: How to help athletes perform and thrive under pressure*. New York, NY: Routledge.

Henriksen, K., Schinke, R. J., McCann, S., Durand-Bush, N., Moesch, K., Parham, W. D., Larsen, C. H., Cogan, K., Donaldsen, A., Poczwardowski, A., Noce, F., & Hunziker, J. (2020). Athlete mental health in the Olympic/Paralympic quadrennium: A multi-societal consensus statement. *International Journal of Sport and Exercise Psychology 18*, 391–408.

Henriksen, K., Schinke, R. J., Moesch, K., McCann, S., Parham, W. D., Larsen, C. H., & Terry, P. (2019). Consensus statement on improving the mental health of high-performance athletes. *International Journal of Sport and Exercise Psychology*. https://doi.org/10.1080/1612197X.2019.1570473.

Ivarsson, A., Stenling, A., Fallby, J., Johnson, U., Borg, E., & Johansson, G. (2015). The predictive ability of the talent development environment on youth elite football players' well-being: A person-centered approach. *Psychology of Sport and Exercise 16*, 15–23.

Jahoda, M. (1958). *Current concepts of positive mental health*. New York: Basic Books.

Jorm, A. F., Korten, A. E., Jacomb, P. A., Christensen, H., Rodgers, B., & Pollitt, P. (1997). Mental health literacy: A survey of the public's ability to recognise mental disorders and their beliefs about the effectiveness of treatment. *The Medical Journal of Australia* 166(4), 166–182.

Joy, E., Kussman, A., & Nattiv, A. (2016). 2016 update on eating disorders in athletes: A comprehensive narrative review with a focus on clinical assessment and management. *British Journal of Sports Medicine 50*, 154–162. doi: 10.1136/bjsports-2015–095735.

Kenttä, G., Hassmen, P., & Raglin, J. (2006). Mood state monitoring of training and recovery in elite kayakers. *European Journal of Sport Science 6*, 245–253. doi: 10.1080/17461390601012652.

Kessler, R. C., Adler, L., Ames, M., Demler, O., Faraone, S., Hiripi, E., ... Walters, E. E. (2005). The world health organization adult ADHD self-report scale (ASRS): A short screening scale for use in the general population. *Psychological Medicine 35*, 245–256. doi: 10.1017/s0033291704002892.

Keyes, C. L. (2002). The mental health continuum: From languishing to flourishing in life. *Journal of Health and Social Behavior 43*, 207–222.

Keyes, C. L. (2007). Promoting and protecting mental health as flourishing: A complementary strategy for improving national mental health. *American Psychologist 62*, 95–108.

Kuettel, A., & Larsen, C. H. (2019). Risk and protective factors for mental health in elite athletes: A scoping review, *International Review of Sport and Exercise Psychology*, doi:10.1080/1750984X.2019.1689574.

Kuettel, A., Boyle, E., & Schmid, J. (2017). Factors contributing to the quality of the transition out of elite sports in Swiss, Danish, and Polish athletes. *Psychology of Sport and Exercise 29*, 27–39.

Kussman, J. E., & Nattiv, A. (2016). 2016 update on eating disorders in athletes: A comprehensive narrative review with a focus on clinical assessment and management. British Journal of Sports Medicine *2016*(50), 154–162. doi:10.1136/bjsports-2015-095735.

Lebrun, F., & Collins, D. (2017). Is elite sport (really) bad for you? Can we answer the question? *Frontiers in Psychology 8*, 324. http://dx.doi.org/10.3389/fpsyg.2017. 00324.

McCann, S., Henriksen, K., Larsen, C. H., Cogan, K., Donaldson, A., Durand-Bush, N., Hunziker, J., Moesch, K., Noce, F., Parham, W. D., & Poczwardowski, A. (2020). Mental health and the games: Developing support strategies for the unique world of Olympic and Paralympic athletes, *The International Society of Sport Psychology* (ISSP).

Mitchell, T. O., Nesti, M., Richardson, D., Midgley, A. W., Eubank, M., & Littlewood, M. (2014). Exploring athletic identity in elite-level youth football: A cross-sectional approach. *Journal of Sports Sciences 32*, 1294–1299. doi: http://dx.doi.org/10.1080/02640414.2014.898855.

Moesch, K., Kenttä, G., Kleinert, J., Quignon-Fleuret, C., Cecil, S., & Bertollo, M. (2018). FEPSAC position statement: Mental health disorders in elite athletes and models of service provision. *Psychology of Sport and Exercise 38*, 61–71.

Morgan, W. P. (1979). Anxiety reduction following acute physical activity. *Psychiatric Annals 9*, 36–45.

Mountjoy, M., Rhind, D. J. A., Tilvas, A., & Leglise, M. (2015). Safeguarding the child athlete in sport: A review, a framework and recommendations for the IOC youth athlete development model. *British Journal of Sports Medicine 49*, 883–886. doi: 10.1136/bjsports-2015–094619.

Murphy, H. B. M. (1978). The meaning of symptom check-list scores in mental health surveys: A testing of multiple hypotheses. *Social Science & Medicine 12*, 67–75.

Nesti, M., & Sully, C. (2014). *Youth development in football lessons from the world's best academies*. London: Routledge.

Park, S., Lavallee, D., & Tod, D. (2013). Athletes' career transition out of sport: A systematic review. *International Review of Sport and Exercise Psychology 6*, 22–53.

Posner, K., Brent, D., Lucas, C., Gould, M., Stanley, B., Brown, G., … Mann, J. (2008). *Columbia-suicide severity rating scale (C-SSRS)*. New York: The Research Foundation for Mental Hygiene. Retrieved from http://cssrs.columbia.edu/wp-content/uploads/C-SSRS1-14-09-Screening.pdf.

Purcell, R., Gwyther, K., & Rice, S. M. (2019). Mental health in elite athletes: Increased awareness requires an early intervention framework to respond to athlete needs. *Sports Medicine – Open*. doi: 10.1186/s40798-019-0220-1.

Putukian, M. (2016). The psychological response to injury in student athletes: A narrative review with a focus on mental health. *British Journal of Sports Medicine 50*, 145–148. doi:10.1136/bjsports-2015–095586.

Raedeke, T. D., & Smith, A. L. (2001). Development and preliminary validation of an athlete burnout measure. *Journal of Sport & Exercise Psychology 23*, 281–306. doi: 10.1123/jsep.23.4.281.

Rancourt, D., Brauer, A., Palermo, M., Choquette, E. M., & Stanley, C. (2019). Response to Tomalski et al. Recommendations for adapting a comprehensive athlete mental health screening program for broad dissemination. *Journal of Sport Psyshology in Action 11*, 57–67. doi: https://doi.org/10.1080/21520704.2020.1722770.

Reardon, C. L., & Factor, R. M. (2010). Sport psychiatry. A systematic review of diagnoses and medical treatment of mental illness in athletes. *Sports Medicine 40*, 961–980. http://dx.doi.org/10.2165/11536580-000000000-00000.

Reardon, C. L., Hainline, B., Aron, C. M., Baron, D., Baum, A. L., Bindra, A., Budgett, R., Campriani, N., Castaldelli-Maia, J. M., Currie, A., Derevensky, J. L., Glick, I. D., Gorczynski, P., Gouttebarge, V., Grandner, M. A., Han, D. H., McDuff, D., Mountjoy, M., Polat, A., … Engebretsen, L. (2019). Mental health in elite athletes: International Olympic Committee consensus statement. *British Journal of Sports Medicine 53*, 667–699. http://doi.org/10.1136/bjsports-2019-100715.

Reinboth, M., & Duda, J. L. (2006). Perceived motivational climate need satisfaction and indices of well-being in team sports: A longitudinal perspective. *Psychology of Sport and Exercise* 7, 269–286. doi: 10.1016/j.psychsport.2005.06.002.

Rice, S. M., Purcell, R., De Silva, S., Mawren, D., McGorry, P. D., & Parker, A. G. (2016). The mental health of elite athletes: A narrative systematic review. *Sports Medicine 46*, 1333–1353.

Rice, S. M., Parker, A. G., Mawren, D., Clifton, P., Harcourt, P., Lloyd, M., Kountouris, A., Smith, B., McGorry, P. D., & Purcell, R. (2019). Preliminary psychometric validation of a brief screening tool for athlete mental health among male elite athletes: The Athlete Psychological Strain Questionnaire. *International Journal of Sport and Exercise Psychology*. doi: https://doi.org/10.1080/1612197X.2019.1611900.

Ryff, C. D. (1989). "Happiness is everything, or is it? Explorations on the meaning of psychological well-being." *Journal of Personality and Social Psychology 57,* 1069–1081. doi:10.1037/0022-3514.57.6.1069.

Samuels, C., James, L., Lawson, D., & Meeuwisse, W. (2016). The Athlete sleep screening questionnaire: A new tool for assessing and managing sleep in elite athletes. *British Journal of Sports Medicine 50*, 418–422. doi:10.1136/bjsports-2014-0944332.

Schaal, K., Tafflet, M., Nassif, H., Thibault, V., Pichard, C., Alcotte, M., … Uddin, M. (2011). Psychological balance in high level athletes: Gender-based differences and sport-specific patterns. *PLoS ONE, 6*(5): 319007. doi:10.1371/journal.pone.0019007.

Schinke, R. J., Stambulova, N. B., Si, G., & Moore, Z. (2017). International society of sport psychology position stand: Athletes' mental health, performance, and development. *International Journal of Sport and Exercise Psychology 16*, 1–18.

Skinner, H. A. (1982). The drug abuse screening test. Addictive Behavior 7(4), 363–371. doi: 10.1016/0306-4603(82)90005-3.

Slingerland, K. V., Durand-Bush, N., & Rathwell, S. (2018). Levels and prevalence of mental health functioning in Canadian university student-athletes. *Canadian Journal of Higher Education 48*, 149–168. doi: 10.7202/1057108ar.

Souter, G., Lewis, R., & Serrant, L. (2018). Men, mental health and elite sport: A narrative review. *Sports Medicine – Open*. doi: 10.1186/s40798-018-0175-7.

Spitzer, R. L., Kroenke, K., & Williams, J. B. W. (1999). Validation and utility of a self-report version of PRIME-MD: The PHQ Primary Care study. *The Journal of the American Medical Association 282*(18), 1737–1744. doi: 10.1001/jama.282.18.1737.

Spitzer, R. L., Kroenke, K., Williams, J. B. W., & Lowe, B. (2006). A brief measure of assessing generalized anxiety disorder. *Archives of Internal Medicine 166*, 1092–1097. doi:10.1001/archinte.166.10.1092.

Storch, E. A., Bagner, D., Merlo, L. J., Shapira, N. A., Geffken, G. R., Murphy, T. K., & Goodman, W. K. (2007). Florida obsessive-compulsive inventory: Development, reliability, and validity. *Journal of Clinical Psychology 63*, 851–859. doi: 10.1002/jclp.20382.

Swann, C. H., Moran, A., & Piggott, D. (2015). Defining elite athletes: Issues in the study of expert performance in sport psychology. *Psychology of Sport and Exercise, 16*, 3–14. http://dx.doi.org/10.1016/j.psychsport.2014.07.004.

Swann, C., Telenta, J., Draper, G., Liddle, S., Fogarty, A., Hurley, D., & Vella, S. (2018). Youth sport as a context for supporting mental health: Adolescent male perspectives. *Psychology of Sport and Exercise 35*, 55–64.

Thiemann, P., Legenbauer, T., Vocks, S., Platen, P., Auyeung, B., & Herpertz, S. (2015). Eating disorders and their putative risk factors among female German professional athletes. *European Eating Disorders Review 23,* 269–276.

Tomalski, J., Clevinger, K., Albert, E., Jackson, R., Wartalowicz, K., & Petrie, T. A. (2019). Mental health screening for athletes: Program development, implementation, and evaluation. *Journal of Sport Psychology in Action 10*, 121–135. doi: 10.1080/21520704.2019.1604589.

Van Slingerland, K., Chin, B., & Durand-Bush, N. (2019, July). Provision of sport-focused mental health care by the CCMHS: Characteristics and mental health challenges of athletes and coaches seeking services. In G. Konttä (Chair), *Mental health in competitive sports: Research and mental health programs from three countries*. Symposium conducted at the 15th European Congress of Sport & Exercise Psychology, Münster, Germany.

Van Slingerland, K. J., Durand-Bush, N., & Kenttä, G. (2019). Collaboratively designing the Canadian centre for mental health and sport (CCMHS) using group concept mapping. *Journal of Applied Sport Psychology*, doi: https://doi.org/10.1080/10413200.2019.1704938.

Walton, M., Murray, E., & Christian, M. D. (2020). Mental health care for medical staff and affiliated healthcare workers during the COVID-19 pandemic. *European Heart Journal: Acute Cardiovascular Care 9*, 241–247. doi: 10.1177/2048872620922795.

World Health Organization (WHO). (2014). *Mental health: A state of well-being*. Geneva, Switzerland: World Health Organization.

PART I

Cases and structures of mental health across countries

2

MENTAL HEALTH IN GERMANY

Examples of good practice in preventing mental disorders and promoting mental health in elite athletes

Marion Sulprizio, Jens Kleinert, and Johanna Belz

Context and conceptual background

In 2009 the German national soccer goalkeeper Robert Enke committed suicide due to severe depression. At the time it was becoming increasingly acknowledged that elite athletes are not protected from or immune to mental health disorders (e.g., depression, burnout, anxiety) but are at the same risk as the normal population (Belz, Kleinert, Ohlert, Rau, & Allroggen, 2018; Frank, Nixdorf, & Beckmann, 2015; Junge & Feddermann-Demont, 2016) or even more prone to specific mental health problems such as eating disorders (Bratland-Sanda & Sundgot-Borgen, 2013). Over the past decade there has been an increasing interest in supporting athletes' mental health (Moesch et al., 2018) and also in Germany the first applied initiatives (e.g., *MentalEmpowerment*, Robert-Enke-Foundation, Department for Sport Psychiatry) providing support for elite athletes with regard to their mental health were founded. These initiatives focus on either the prevention of or therapy for mental health disorders. In order to offer the optimal level of support, athletes should receive help at an early stage in their development so that prevention programs on sport psychology basics (e.g., activation regulation, self-talk, positive imagery) can foster their mental strength or resilience. This becomes important when critical situations like injury, squad selection processes, or stressful personal situations (e.g., exams, conflicts with parents or peers) occur and increase the individual stress level of the athlete. Furthermore, help also should be offered when athletes are already suffering from more severe mental health problems (e.g., depressive mood, anxiety, or eating disorders).

Prevention of mental disorders and promotion of mental health

Working in the area of mental health in athletes covers two different approaches, namely the prevention of mental disorders and the promotion of mental health. The first approach is based on a pathogenetic orientation and aims to change or influence processes that potentially lead to mental disorders. The second approach is based on a salutogenetic orientation (Antonowsky, 1987) and focuses on an athlete's resources to cope with stressors by improving his/her personal and living conditions. Both approaches can be distinguished theoretically;

however, in practice these two concepts go hand in hand. Nevertheless, the theoretical distinction of both concepts is important as it leads to different aims and sometimes even different interventions, strategies, measures, or treatments.

The prevention of mental disorders is typically linked to theoretical models of stress (e.g., transactional model; Lazarus & Folkman, 1984), or other theories that are common in research and explain mental disorders in elite sport (e.g., bio-psycho-social approach; Engel, 1977). Such approaches describe a variety of tasks, affordances, and demands in an athlete's life (e.g., injury, squad selection processes, change of team membership) that are likely to overstrain his or her opportunities to adapt to the given situation and lead to negative outcomes (e.g., depression, anxiety, unhealthy behavior). In athletes, potentially overstraining stressors are related to different contexts (e.g., training, competition, family, and education) and to different relationships and roles in an athlete's life (e.g., team member, opponent, child, spouse, father, and pupil). Avoiding, reducing or weakening overstraining stressors is the core idea of prevention by changing an athlete's environment (e.g., lower physical demands) or by building protective shields against external stressors.

Promotion of mental health focuses on factors that help an individual to remain healthy while facing a stressor that potentially may lead to mental disorders. In salutogenesis (Antonowsky, 1987), these factors are bundled in the sense of coherence (SOC) which is defined as a person's view on his or her own life as being manageable, comprehensible, and meaningful. This sense of coherence is strongly connected to other approaches that define individuals' resources for dealing with problems and stressors (e.g., resilience, hardiness, mental toughness, coping; Eriksson & Lindström, 2006). Therefore, the promotion of mental health means to help individuals to identify, recognize or develop psycho-social factors in an individually harmonious (i.e., accepted and possible) way.

Interrelations between mental health, performance, and personality development

While working with athletes, SPCs are often confronted with the athletes´ desire to improve their performance. But, mental health, performance, and personality development build a triangular holistic picture that has to be considered when planning measures and strategies in the consultation process (FEPSAC, 1995). In this picture, there are two reciprocal paths describing the interplay between mental health and performance or personality development named the mental health-performance path and the mental health-personality path.

Considering the mental health-performance path, it is evident that athletes are striving for a perfect performance, trying to reach challenging goals and presenting their competences in competitions and training situations. Thus, performance is both a requirement and a part of an athlete's identity (Ronkainen, Kavoura, & Ryba, 2016). Therefore, positive or negative changes in performance (e.g., winning, losing, and feeling in or out of shape, injuries) are directly connected to positive or negative changes in mood and emotional dispositions. Hence, from a long-term perspective especially, mental health or well-being can be seen as a fundament for peak performance (Aoyagi, Portenga, Poczwardowski, Cohen, & Statler, 2012; Petitpas & Tinsley, 2014). Conversely, an athlete in a depressed or negative mood is not able to perform in the best possible way (Hanin, 2000).

Considering the mental health- personality path, it is evident that personality development can be defined as the process of change over the lifetime considering various developmental tasks (Havighurst, 1974), which can be general in nature (e.g., establishing a stable identity) or sport-related (e.g., fostering one's athletic career; Ohlert & Ott, 2017). Solving such developmental tasks in a certain sensitive period of learning contributes to positive social feedback, satisfied psychological basic needs (e.g., for relatedness, autonomy, or competence) and, in turn, fosters life satisfaction, mental health, or well-being (Havighurst, 1974). Vice versa, mental health influences personality development in such a way that a mentally healthy person is more capable of solving his or her individual developmental tasks (general or sport-specific).

The mental health-performance path and mental health-personality path can be completed by the interrelation between performance and personality development. Dealing with performance (e.g., success, failure) can be defined as a sport-related developmental task (Ohlert & Ott, 2017). In addition, performance influences social conditions (e.g., member of team) or socio-economic status, which are also important in personality development. Vice versa, personality development contributes to an athlete's performance in such a way that a person who has solved difficult or burdening situations in his or her life can transfer the feelings of success and capability to sport situations and master those in the same way (e.g., general self-efficacy; Bandura, 1977).

The case: Initiatives for mental health in elite sport

Both of the German initiatives described in this chapter address the strongly connected issues of mental disorders and mental health in elite sport and can be considered as good practice examples in Germany for the organization of national or regional sport psychology consulting in order to promote mental health and prevent mental disorders based on a scientific foundation.

mentaltalent: *Sport psychology services for adolescent elite athletes*

mentaltalent is a regional German program which offers systematic and holistic sport psychological support for adolescent elite athletes representing North Rhine-Westphalia (NRW). *mentaltalent* was founded in 2007 at the Institute of Psychology of the GSU, receives funding from the Sport Foundation NRW and closely cooperates with the Olympic training centers, which are responsible for sport psychological services offered to athletes at higher national and international levels.

Structure and aims of mentaltalent

The structure of *mentaltalent* includes a project leader and a project coordinator, who both are affiliated with the Institute of Psychology at the GSU. An expert network consists of 34 SPCs that implement sport psychological services for athletes across NRW and work on a freelance basis for *mentaltalent*. All SPCs are listed on the expert database from the German Federal Institute of Sports Science (BISp) and are qualified by the German Association for Sport Psychology (asp) with a curriculum for applied sport psychology or equivalent qualifications. As the athletic career is only a transitional phase in the life of adolescent elite athletes, *mentaltalent* aims to not only enhance athletes' sport performance but also to support their holistic development. As such, the sport psychological support of *mentaltalent* is based on four pillars: (1) dual career, (2) physical and mental health, (3) development of athletic performance, and (4) personality development.

In order to support athletes in adequately coping with the coinciding demands of their athletic and academic *dual career*, they are supported by *mentaltalent* in analyzing challenges associated with the demands of the various areas of their lives, identifying existing and developing new resources and coping strategies. Furthermore, *mentaltalent* helps athletes to establish a clear overview of their different activities and better organize their time through the formulation of goals and the development of concrete action plans. *Physical and mental health*, both inside and outside of the sport environment, are the foundation of athletic performance and might prevent early career dropout (Schinke, Stambulova, Si, & Moore, 2018). To maintain and promote the mental health of athletes, *mentaltalent* teaches them techniques and strategies to reflect on their own mental and physical state. When the mental health of an athlete is thought to be compromised, additional psychotherapeutic or psychiatric care is made accessible to the athlete by connecting him or her to the German initiative *MentalEmpowerment*. *mentaltalent* supports the *development of athletic performance* and thereby reflects the central goal of many young elite athletes, their coaches, and other stakeholders. To develop their athletic performance, *mentaltalent* supports athletes in learning psychological skills training (PST) techniques and strategies. PST is an educational approach in which psychological skills such as imagery, relaxation, and self-talk are viewed as learnable (Vealey, 1988). *mentaltalent* promotes athletes' *personality development* by helping them to understand the roles that they occupy in different life contexts (e.g., in school, in their teams, in their families). The awareness about and reflection on these different – and sometimes conflicting – roles helps athletes to understand expectations, responsibilities, and rights associated with these roles. Furthermore, the acquisition and improvement of social competencies plays an important role in the personality development of athletes so they learn strategies to enhance self-confidence, self-efficacy, self-reflection, conflict resolution abilities, tolerance, and communication skills.

Sport psychology services by mentaltalent

Since its foundation in 2007, *mentaltalent* has offered a variety of sport psychological services to athletes, coaches, and sport boarding school staff. Services for athletes consist of group workshops and individual sport psychology consulting, services for coaches consist of group supervisions, case reviews, and individual consulting ('coach-the-coach'), and services for sport boarding schools consist of sport psychological consultation hours for athletes and individual consulting for the leading staff of the boarding schools. To ensure the quality of the services offered, the SPCs belonging to the expert-network can participate in intervisions organized by *mentaltalent*. These intervisions, defined as a collegial counseling service in psychosocial professions (Wylleman, 2019), are offered six times a year with the aim of exchanging experiences and discussing cases under the supervision of a licensed supervisor. The services offered for athletes, coaches, and sport boarding school staff are framed by a sport psychological diagnostic process and a standardized evaluation. *mentaltalent* offers a variety of group workshops for clubs and federations, each lasting from 1.5 to 2.5 hours. The majority of workshop topics can be categorized into five modules: "Motivation, emotion & stress," "Performing under pressure," "Life and sport skills," "Communication and self-confidence," and "Team success." The workshops are conducted using the didactic method of peer teaching (Topping, 2005), which is based on the assumption that athletes are experts in their own sport, feelings, and experiences. Therefore, athletes are encouraged to share their feelings, experiences, and coping strategies with other athletes during the workshops. The workshop leader's task is to guide and moderate the exchange of information. Workshop topics are progressively added to *mentaltalent*'s workshop-portfolio based on intensive communication with SPCs in order to identify needs of athletes, coaches, and staff of sport boarding schools. Currently, *mentaltalent* offers 30 workshop topics. To ensure high quality workshop content, *mentaltalent* provides SPCs with theory-based content-outlines, worksheets, and handouts for each workshop topic. Since *mentaltalent*'s foundation, the demand for group workshops has increased drastically from ten delivered workshops in the year 2007 to 175 delivered workshops in 2019. Simultaneously, the number of participants has grown from approximately 150 in 2007 to over 4000 supported athletes from 2007 until the end of 2019.

Another sport psychology service offered by *mentaltalent* is individual sport psychology consulting. In this individual consulting process, which usually includes six sessions of 60 minutes each, personal challenges and issues are worked on in a more systematic and in-depth manner than the group workshop format. The central goal of the individual sport psychology consulting is that athletes reflect and better understand their own behaviors and roles in a systemic context (e.g., considering the different relationships and roles in their lives). With this understanding, athletes can identify resources, recognize potentials, and deduce strengths and action strategies in order to tackle personal challenges. In 2019, 85 athletes received individual sport psychology consulting compared to only eight athletes in 2007.

Diagnostic process and evaluation in mentaltalent

A sport psychological diagnostic process frames every individual sport psychology consulting. Before the first and after the fifth consulting session, a sport psychological diagnostic assesses several intra- and interpersonal factors. Intrapersonal factors refer to motivational, volitional, and emotional variables, the utilization of mental techniques, sport-related self-efficacy, physical and mental well-being, and coping resources. With regard to interpersonal factors, social support, team cohesion, and need satisfaction are investigated. In addition to the issues and challenges that are personally communicated by the athlete, the results of the diagnostic investigation give the SPC and the athlete important indications for potential areas of improvement. The results of the post-diagnostic, on the other hand, provide information as to whether the areas identified for improvement were developed during the course of the individual consulting. After the completion of every individual sport psychology service, participants are invited to evaluate this on a voluntary basis. In order to receive structured feedback, *mentaltalent* uses the QS17 (Kleinert & Ohlert, 2014), which covers the perceived quality of the consulting situation, the perceived improvement in psychosocial abilities or skills, and the perceived impact of the consulting on athletes' performance and personal development.

MentalEmpowerment*: Network initiative for mental health in elite sport*

The German nationwide network initiative "*MentalEmpowerment* – mental health in elite sport" was founded in 2011 as an institution at the Institute of Psychology at the GSU.

Structure and aims of MentalEmpowerment

MentalEmpowerment follows the aim to maintain and promote mental health in elite sport. Additionally, a concern of *MentalEmpowerment* is to prevent psychological problems, such as excessive stress, depression or burnout in elite sport, and to provide contacts for the right treatment. At the center of *MentalEmpowerment*'s structure is the *coordination center* (see Figure 2.1), which is responsible for the management of emerging processes and for the scientific direction. Managing the processes means coordinating the current business, implementing decisions, and maintaining a network of SPCs, psychotherapists, and psychiatrists. The scientific direction ensures the integration of a scientific perspective as well as holding the administrative supervision of the management.

The content-based orientation of *MentalEmpowerment* is provided by a *steering group* that consists of six renowned experts with sport psychological, psychotherapeutic or psychiatric expertise, which ensures an interdisciplinary exchange on the subject of mental health in elite sport in the initiative. The steering group deals with shaping the strategic and innovative orientation of *MentalEmpowerment* and decides on activities that should be organized or developed by the coordination center. The *advisory board* consists of the financial sponsors of the initiative, which comprise the German insurance company for professional athletes, the Robert-Enke-Foundation and the Labor Union of professional soccer players. Based on internal regulations the advisory board discusses and recommends specific projects to implement the tasks of *MentalEmpowerment*. One core instrument of *MentalEmpowerment* is a network of SPCs, psychotherapists, and psychiatrists, consisting of more than 300 experts. The network primarily functions as a database of specialist partners in cases where athletes need additional help (e.g., sport psychology consulting or therapy). The high number of network partners and the nationwide distribution guarantee that an appropriate intervention can be arranged quickly near to the home of an athlete. The work and tasks of *MentalEmpowerment* can be categorized into four working areas (see Figure 2.1): "counseling and referral," "information and public relations," "further education and events," and "early detection and screening."

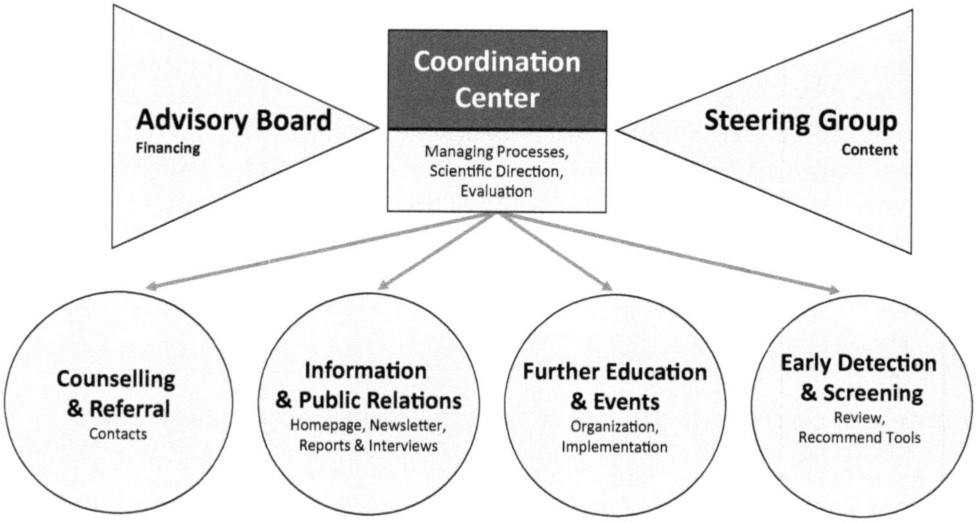

FIGURE 2.1 Structure and working areas of *MentalEmpowerment*

Counseling and referral

Athletes, as well as coaches, parents, or SPCs can contact the coordination center of *MentalEmpowerment* when they are seeking help for mental health related issues. Within an initial exploratory talk, *MentalEmpowerment* determines which form of support should be offered to the athlete (i.e., sport psychology consulting or therapy). In a second step, the coordination center provides 2–3 contacts (including addresses, professional title, email addresses, phone numbers, websites) from the nationwide network. The network partners guarantee prompt care and treatment close to home. The SPCs are members of an expert database from the German Federal Institute of Sports Science (BISp) and are qualified according to a curriculum offered by the German Association for Sport Psychology (asp) or an equivalent qualification. The therapists are members of German psychotherapeutic or psychiatric unions and are additionally qualified in the field of elite sport. The selection of a suitable expert is managed by the coordination center of *MentalEmpowerment* via a digital network map of Germany, on which the regional distribution of the network partners is registered. The network of experts consists of 346 persons (170 SPCs, 77 psychotherapists, 61 psychiatrists, and 38 from other professions like pedagogy). From 2011 to 2019, *MentalEmpowerment* delivered mental health-related services to 454 athletes (200 male, 227 female, and 27 not specified) from various sport disciplines. Consulting concerns ranged from subclinical concerns (e.g., choking under pressure, dealing with injuries, managing mistakes and defeats) to suspected clinical concerns (e.g., depressed mood, suicidal thoughts, anxiety, suspected eating disorders, suspected sport addiction). Three weeks after submitting contact dates to athletes, the coordination center sends an "aftercare" email in which each athlete is asked about his or her well-being and his or her satisfaction with the provided contacts. In most cases athletes report that they are satisfied and have been able to make contact with a suitable SPC, psychotherapist, or psychiatrist. If athletes still need help or want to change the therapist, *MentalEmpowerment* offers contact information for appropriate experts. This process is continued until the athlete feels that he or she is in "good hands."

Information and public relations

MentalEmpowerment aims at disseminating knowledge about mental health in elite sports in order to enhance health literacy and to prevent stigmatization in the population. To achieve this, *MentalEmpowerment* provides information on the topic of "mental health in elite sport" to different target groups by different approaches that have been developed over the course of the past years. One approach is participation in lectures, talks, and publications. Current information on the topic of "mental health in elite sport" is also distributed via the website www.mentalempowerment.de which offers information about the development of the initiative, a comprehensive bibliography, a current press review, research news, and best practice examples. Additionally, a flyer – available in German and English – provides information about the goals and services offered by the initiative. This flyer is distributed in Olympic training centers, sport boarding schools, and the expert network. Furthermore, every six months a newsletter about current initiative developments and offers is sent to everyone in the expert network. Finally, *MentalEmpowerment* defines itself as an information and contact portal for all kinds of media inquiries (e.g., print media, radio, and television) and cooperates with these media partners via interview.

Further education and events

MentalEmpowerment promotes knowledge and competence in the field of mental health and mental illness in elite sport by various educational means (e.g., topic-specific symposia, further education courses, lectures) and for different target groups (e.g., athletes, coaches/trainers, SPCs, psychotherapists). Since its foundation, *MentalEmpowerment* has organized and carried out four large symposia on the topic of mental health in elite sport and was responsible for ten further education programs (e.g., prevention of mental health problems, promotion of mental health by sport psychological workshops, prevention of sexual violence, dealing with traumatic situations and injuries).

Screening and early detection

Over the years *MentalEmpowerment* has developed a screening process when athletes in other sport psychology programs such as *mentaltalent* address the GSU for standardized sport psychological diagnostics (e.g., self-efficacy, emotional control, group cohesion), including screening for impaired psychological well-being (WHO-5; World Health Organization, 1998), and depressive mood (PHQ-2; Kroenke, Spitzer, & Williams, 2003). If critical values are detected (i.e., falling below or exceeding certain cut offs) *MentalEmpowerment* contacts the athlete (and his/her parents) via email and offers different support options (e.g., contact to psychotherapeutic or psychiatric care).

Interplay between mentaltalent *and* MentalEmpowerment

mentaltalent and *MentalEmpowerment* complement each other in terms of their target groups, covered issues, and services offered. The adolescent elite athletes from the *mentaltalent* program have the opportunity to benefit from the services of *MentalEmpowerment* concerning mental health issues. *mentaltalent* delivers a wide range of services for young elite athletes including performance enhancement, personality development, mental health and dual career issues while *MentalEmpowerment* focuses on mental health issues. For that reason, athletes from *mentaltalent* can take advantage of services provided by *MentalEmpowerment* and, for example, benefit from psychotherapy referral at short notice. The expert networks of *mentaltalent* and *MentalEmpowerment* are functionally overlapping and complementary to each other. The expert partners of *mentaltalent* are mainly located in NRW, while *MentalEmpowerment* uses a nationwide network to refer athletes from all over Germany to an appropriate expert. As the network of *MentalEmpowerment* consists of experts in the professions of sport psychology, psychotherapy, and psychiatry, athletes from *mentaltalent* have access to all of the aforementioned professions and services. Both initiatives follow similar standards of qualification for their experts in that the network partners have to meet certain qualification requirements in order to participate in the networks of *mentaltalent* or *MentalEmpowerment* (e.g., criteria of the Federal Institute of Sports Science or the German psychotherapeutic and psychiatric union). *mentaltalent* and *MentalEmpowerment* further cooperate when dealing with incoming requests. If it becomes necessary for athletes in the *mentaltalent* program to receive psychotherapeutic or psychiatric help for clinical mental health disorders, these athletes are referred to *MentalEmpowerment* for the subsequent process of finding an appropriate expert for these athletes. Conversely, *MentalEmpowerment* refers to *mentaltalent* when an athlete is located in

NRW and is searching for sport psychological support. *mentaltalent* and *MentalEmpowerment* are further linked in terms of early detection and screening because *mentaltalent's* standardized sport psychological diagnostic process (e.g., self-efficacy, emotional control, group cohesion) also includes a screening for impaired psychological well-being and depressive mood. *MentalEmpowerment* offers contact to psychotherapists or psychiatrists when the screening data indicate a serious mental disorder.

The cooperation between *mentaltalent* and *MentalEmpowerment* can be described as a good practice example of holistic care for adolescent elite athletes and should be pursued in the future.

Reflections

In Germany, there is a noticeable positive tendency toward the de-stigmatization of mental health problems in sport. More and more stakeholders in the field of elite sport understand that mental health disorders such as depression, anxiety, and eating disorders are usual to some degree and have to be prevented, addressed, or treated. Additionally, they understand that mental health problems do not have to result in drop out from elite sport and that it is not a sign of weakness to suffer from a mental health disorder. Similar to severe physical injuries, athletes need time to recover and to return to competition after a mental health problem. Thus, as a recommendation for future endeavors in Germany and also in other countries the information process about mental health and mental disorders in elite sport should be fostered to fight against the stigmatization. For this reason, initiatives like *mentaltalent* and *MentalEmpowerment* should be supported or expanded by national funding. Resources (in terms of finance and personnel) should be enhanced, networks should be expanded, and regional programs (i.e., *mentaltalent*) should be transferred to other federal states or other countries in response to the increasing number of elite athletes that are searching for sport psychological or therapeutic help to prevent or treat a mental health disorder.

A further perspective for Germany and other countries should be an improvement in the collaboration between different professions (sport psychology, psychotherapy, psychiatry) that are active in the field of mental health in elite sport. Specifically, the roles of different professions should be clarified as this clarity seems to be the basis for cooperation and, ultimately achieving the common goal of supporting athletes. Another means to facilitate optimal cooperation is the generation of a positive climate in the group of different professions. This positive climate can be supported by a trusting relationship with each other, by taking advantage of opportunities to discuss current problems at an early stage and, furthermore, by jointly contributing to the mental health of athletes. Moreover, the climate within different professions should be shaped by a positive communication, respect, and mutual appreciation. In Germany, there are already mutual symposia and events for all of the aforementioned professions (e.g., events organized by *MentalEmpowerment* or the German Association for Psychiatry, Psychotherapy and Psychosomatics) that provide the opportunity for exchange, collaboration, and network building. Additionally, textbooks and publications on the topic of mental health in elite sport should jointly be edited by experts of different professions, which highlight the legitimacy of all participants in this important field.

Furthermore, the international collaboration on the topic of mental health in elite sport should be fostered. The German initiatives conduct cooperation, meetings, and discussions with organizations and programs of other countries (e.g., Swedish School of Sport and Health

Sciences, Swiss Association of Sport Psychology) what is considered as a relevant step to improve in the field of mental health in elite sport. Such constructive exchanges intend to contribute to a worldwide attitude change and, therefore, the further de-stigmatization of the field of mental health in elite sport.

In the future, the initiatives *mentaltalent* and *MentalEmpowerment*, with their networks of scientists and practitioners from sport psychology, psychotherapy, and psychiatry, should more intensively discuss the common goals and programs that contribute to the mental health of athletes. This could be a further step in learning from other countries and sharing strategies that have already been developed.

References

Antonovsky, A. (1987). *Unraveling the mystery of health: How people manage stress and stay well.* San Francisco: Jossey-Bass.

Aoyagi, M. W., Portenga, S. T., Poczwardowski, A., Cohen, A. B., & Statler, T. (2012). Reflections and directions: The profession of sport psychology past, present, and future. *Professional Psychology: Research and Practice 43*(1), 32–38. doi:10.1037/a0025676.

Bandura, A. (1977). Self-efficacy: Toward a unifying theory of behavioral change. *Psychological Review 84*(2), 191–215. doi:10.1016/0146-6402(78)90009-7.

Belz, J., Kleinert, J., Ohlert, J., Rau, T., & Allroggen, M. (2018). Risk for depression and psychological well-being in German national and state team athletes: Associations with age, gender, and performance level. *Journal of Clinical Sport Psychology 12*(2), 160–178. doi:10.1123/jcsp.2016-0024.

Bratland-Sanda, S., & Sundgot-Borgen, J. (2013). Eating disorders in athletes: Overview of prevalence, risk factors and recommendations for prevention and treatment. *European Journal of Sport Science 13*(5), 499–508. doi:10.1080/17461391.2012.740504.

Engel, G. L. (1977). The need for a new medical model: A challenge for biomedicine. *Science 196*(4286), 129–136. doi:10.1126/science.847460.

Eriksson, M., & Lindström, B. (2006). Antonovsky's sense of coherence scale and the relation with health: A systematic review. *Journal of Epidemiology and Community Health 60*(5), 376–381. doi:10.1136/jech.2005.041616.

FEPSAC (1995). *Position statements – 1.Definition of sport psychology, 1995.* Retrieved from www.fepsac.com/activities/position_statements/

Frank, R., Nixdorf, I., & Beckmann, J. (2015). Depression among elite athletes: Prevalence and psychological factors. *Deutsche Zeitschrift für Sportmedizin 64,* 320–329.

Hanin, Y. L. (2000). Individual Zones of Optimal Functioning (IZOF) model. In Y. L. Hanin (Ed.), *Emotions in Sport* (pp. 65–89). Champaign: Human Kinetics.

Havighurst, R. J. (1974). *Developmental tasks and education* (3rd ed.). New York: McKay.

Junge, A., & Feddermann-Demont, N. (2016). Prevalence of depression and anxiety in top-level male and female football players. *BMJ Open Sport & Exercise Medicine,* (2), 1–7. doi:10.1136/bmjsem-2015-000087.

Junge, A., & Prinz, B. (2019). Depression and anxiety symptoms in 17 teams of female football players including 10 German first league teams. *British Journal of Sports Medicine 53*(8), 471–477. doi:10.1136/bjsports-2017-098033.

Kleinert, J., & Ohlert, J. (2014). Ergebnisqualität in der sportpsychologischen Beratung und Betreuung: Konstruktion und erste Ergebnisse des Befragungsinventars QS17. *Zeitschrift für Sportpsychologie 21*(1), 13–22. doi:10.1026/1612-5010/a000110

Kroenke, K., Spitzer, R. L., & Williams, J. B. (2003). The patient health questionnaire-2: Validity of a two-item depression screener. *Medical Care 41,* 1284–1294.

Lazarus, R. S., & Folkman, S. (1984). *Stress, appraisal, and coping.* New York: Springer.

Moesch, K., Janttä, G., Kleinert, J., Quignon-Fleuret, C., Cecil, S., & Bertollo, M. (2018). FEPSAC position statement: Mental health disorders in elite athletes and models of service provision. *Psychology of Sport and Exercise 38,* 61–71. doi:10.1016/j.psychsport.2018.05.013.

Nixdorf, I., Frank, R., Hautzinger, M., & Beckmann, J. (2013). Prevalence of depressive symptoms and correlating variables among German elite athletes. *Journal of Clinical Sport Psychology* 7(4), 313–326.

Ohlert, J., & Ott, I. (2017). Developmental tasks and well-being in adolescent elite athletes in comparison with recreational/non-athletes. *European Journal of Sports Science.* doi:10.1080/17461391.2017.1365935.

Petitpas, A. J., & Tinsley, T. M. (2014). Counseling interventions in applied sport psychology. In J. L. van Raalte & B. W. Brewer (Eds.), *Exploring sport and exercise psychology* (pp. 241–259). Washington, D.C.: American Psychological Association.

Ronkainen, N. J., Kavoura, A., & Ryba, T. V. (2016). A meta-study of athletic identity research in sport psychology: Current status and future directions. *International Review of Sport and Exercise Psychology 9*(1), 45–64. doi:10.1080/1750984X.2015.1096414.

Schinke, R. J., Stambulova, N. B., Si, G., & Moore, Z. (2018). International society of sport psychology position stand: Athletes' mental health, performance, and development. *International Journal of Sport and Exercise Psychology 16*(6), 622–639. doi:10.1080/1612197X.2017.1295557.

Topping, K. J. (2005). Trends in peer learning. *International Journal of Experimental Educational Psychology 25*(6), 631–645.

Vealey, R. S. (1988). Future directions in psychological skills training. *The Sport Psychologist 2,* 318–336.

World Health Organization (1998). *Use of well-being measures in primary health care – the DepCare project health for all: Target 12. E60246.* Psychiatric Research Unit. Geneva, Switzerland: WHO.

World Health Organization (2004). *Promoting mental health: Concepts, emerging evidence, practice.* A report of the World Health Organization. Geneva: World Health Organization.

Wylleman, P. (2019). An organizational perspective on applied sport psychology in elite sport. Psychology of Sport and Exercise *42,* 89–99.

3

MENTAL HEALTH IN ELITE SPORT

Perspectives from sub-Saharan Africa

Tshepang Tshube, Lingani Mbakile-Mahlanza, Gaorekwe V. Nthutang, and Justice Dipeba

Background: Elite athletes in sub-Saharan Africa

Africa is the second largest continent with most of its countries recording low income levels (Akachi & Canning, 2007), high prevalence of communicable diseases (Novitsky et al., 2018), high corruption rates (Ford et al., 2011) and high levels of unemployed youth (Ackah-Baidoo, 2016;). The sub-Saharan region has been experiencing the youth bulge. Lin (2012) defined the youth bulge as a steady increase in the youth population thus making them the largest share of the country population.Youth adults in the sub-Saharan region constitute over 10% of the global population in the 15–49 age category (Abu-Raddad et al., 2013). These social and demographic factors play a pivotal role in influencing public health outcomes. For example, the 2018 World Health Organization report indicates that the African region is the most HIV affected, with almost 1 in every 25 adults (3.9%) living with HIV and comprising of over two-thirds of the people living with HIV globally. These are some of the major challenges sub-Saharan leaders have to address.

In light of these challenges, mental health issues receive very little attention from policy makers and governments across the African continent (Gureje & Alem, 2000). In fact, governments in sub-Saharan Africa spend significantly less on mental health (about 1%) compared to spending on infections and other related illnesses (Crick, 2010). It is therefore important to recognize that the development of mental health policies and interventions in Africa is closely related to the general social welfare of communities across sub-Saharan Africa (Gureje & Alem, 2000). It is practically impossible to isolate elite athletes' mental health issues from the general social welfare, health, and political issues affecting the sub-Saharan region. The purpose of this chapter is to provide knowledge about mental health issues affecting elite athletes in the sub-Saharan region. The chapter first presents elite athletes' mental health issues in sub-Saharan Africa, followed by socio-cultural and spiritual issues in sports, interventions for mental health issues in sub-Saharan elite sport, and summary as well as recommendations. We reviewed academic literature, used field notes from consultations with athletes, and consulted newspaper reports. It is impossible to have a single view that represents all the 54 sub-Saharan countries hence we will discuss common cases observed across the continent.

The sub-Saharan sport context

Sport and games have an in-depth pre-and post-colonial history in sub-Saharan Africa (Amusa & Toriola, 2010). Research in sub-Saharan Africa indicates that leaders in post-colonial Africa used sport to build national culture, unity, nationhood, recognition, and pan African solidarity. This is evidenced by the 1965 first edition of All-Africa games hosted in Brazzaville, Congo. These games were preceded by the formation of the Organization of African Unity in 1963. Baker (1987) noted that African athletes became international ambassadors and powerful symbols of heroism and national identity. Major sporting events provided African athletes with unique opportunities to earn national and global exposure. Sport in Africa has significantly transformed from the first edition of All African games to African countries competing for gold medals at the summer Olympic games. For example, Batswana, Kenyan, South African, and Ethiopian athletes are some of the most competitive at major international track and field games (e.g., Olympic and world championships). Thus, pressure to win is not exclusive to athletes in industrialized nations. Elite athletes in the sub-Saharan region arguably experience more pressure than elite athletes from other regions. Elite athletes in the sub-Saharan region have fewer resources to prepare for major games, mostly compete and train in alien environment (e.g., Europe and America), and their livelihoods may depend exclusively on their athletic performance. One of Botswana's top track athletes at the Olympics 400 m finals (games withheld) experienced high levels of anxiety and pressure to win caused by his/her interaction with a senior government official (i.e., Minister responsible for sports). The senior government official approached the athlete at the warm-up area minutes before the race and handed the athlete the Botswana national flag and said to the athlete "This is a gold medal I am giving you. Return the flag as a gold medal." Ministers are highly respected and revered in Botswana. The authority figure in the minister certainly put a lot of pressure on the athlete. The athlete, who was a strong medal contender, did not win any medal. When interviewed following the race, the athlete expressed his/her level of anxiety, fear, and frustrations relating to the event. The lack of knowledge and pressure from government officials are some of the challenges sub-Saharan athletes navigate at major games.

Sub-Saharan elite athletes competing at major games have attracted additional incentives beyond national heroism and patriotism. For example, a huge number of sub-Saharan elite athletes have contracts with major sponsors such as Nike, Adidas, and Puma. These contracts have raised elite athletes' "financial appetite" in bonuses and appearance fees, which most countries in the region cannot afford. Elite athletes' need for financial incentives juxtaposed with patriotism and nationality defection are some of the most contested issues in the sub-Saharan sports fraternity (Adjaye, 2010; Peart, 2005). Even though athletes from the sub-Saharan region compete pound for pound with all other international athletes at major games, studies indicate that they struggle to have access to basic social services and health care. A seething problem of lack of compensation, unfair treatment, corruption, and poor training facilities are some of the most cited challenges facing elite athletes in the sub-Saharan region (Agbo, 2019). These issues certainly have a significant impact on athletes' mental state and may distract elite athletes' performance. As they can be seen as stressors, they certainly also influence athletes' mental health.

Newspaper reports in a number of countries in the sub-Saharan region, including Ghana, Kenya, and Nigeria indicate that on several occasions, athletes boycott games in protest of unpaid allowances, lack of proper games attire, and athletes' funds siphoned by officials. Three top Kenyan officials were arrested at the 2016 Olympic games for allegedly siphoning athletes' funds (France-Presse, 2016). It is very complex for a sport psychologist to address such issues at the games. The demands and challenges placed on elite athletes in the sub-Saharan region are unique and severe for any athlete competing at major international games. These challenges and demands exacerbate their susceptibility to mental health problems and risky behaviors.

Elite athletes' mental health issues in sub-Saharan Africa

The limited research on mental health, inadequate mental health services and particularly for elite athletes is severe in the sub-Saharan region. Psychologists (e.g., sport and counseling psychologists) are often invited to consult with athletes and the entire team in preparation for major games. For example, Philomena Balo Ikulayo (1948–2016) was one of the first sub-Saharan sport psychologist to consult with a national team at the Olympic games (Serpa & Stambulova, 2016). She consulted with the 1988, Nigerian team at the Seoul Olympic games. Other sub-Saharan sport psychologists who served at more recent Olympic games include Clinton Gahwiler (team South Africa at the 2004 Athens Olympic games), and Tshepang Tshube (team Botswana at the 2016 Rio Olympic games). Their role is primarily performance enhancement through the development of mental skills training programs. In addition, psychologists conduct team building activities and attend to any social and in rare cases mental health issues in the team (Tshube & Hanrahan, 2016). The most notable observations sport psychologists have to address include mental health issues, socio-cultural issues, and spiritual issues relating to elite athletes' health and sports performance. One of Ikulayo's observations in Nigeria include athletes chanting songs, incarnations, and the use of juju for performance enhancement (Ikulayo & Semidara, 2011). These observations are not unique to Nigeria but common in the sub-Saharan countries.

One of the authors experienced a complex case that involved two coaches and an athlete who were dealing with a "spiritual revelation" in the team. Coach Mazebe (pseudonym) had been appointed to work and travel with the team to one of the major games. Coach Mazebe had a "spiritual revelation" that one of the top athletes would be injured at the games. Following the revelation, Caoch Mazebe informed the concerned athlete about the "revelation" and possible rituals needed to avert the likely injury. Unfortunately, Coach Mazebe could not perform the rituals and also travel with the team due to scheduling conflicts. Coach Tabona (pseudonym) was appointed to replace the previous coach and travel with the team. Upon arrival, the athlete was hesitant to train, compete, and socialize with the rest of the team. The coach then referred the athlete to the medical team for assessment. During the assessment, the medical team observed that the athlete was hesitant to participate in the assessment. Regardless of the hesitation, the assessment was successfully completed, and the results did not reveal any signs of physical injury. Upon further inquiry and psychological assessment, the athlete informed the psychologist of the "revelation" and that the newly appointed coach was aware and had been giving the athlete his own charm/juju/muti to avert the injury. These complexities require deep cultural competence, trust, and good rapport between the coach, athlete, and psychologist. The example also indicates the extent to which athletes and coaches use juju/muti/charm and spiritual revelations in sub-Saharan Africa.

Gureje and Alem (2000) noted that people in Africa strongly believe that mental illness are caused and can be treated through traditional and supernatural powers. Evidence based research and systematic review of literature in Africa and other parts of the world indicates a strong influence of indigenous culture in sport psychology practice (Hagan Jr. & Schack,

2017) and mental health (Hernández et al., 2017). In Ethiopia, there is strong culture of traditional healing and indigenous knowledge. In a study conducted in 1995, Alem, Desta, and Araya noted that about 85% of emotionally disturbed patients had consulted a traditional healer. In a more recent study (Selamu et al., 2015) conducted in Ethiopia, over 150 traditional healers were recorded in rural communities and are considered a strong community resource for health. Even though there is no evidence known to the authors of this chapter that elite athletes in Ethiopia use traditional healers for mental health, it is a reasonable assumption that they practice their culture and often seek medical support from traditional healers.

Socio-cultural and spiritual issues in sub-Saharan sports

Mental health professionals in sub-Saharan Africa sports engage with clients from a culturally diverse society. Uniquely for low-income countries and the sub-Saharan region, there is a huge population of professionals who are not native to the region. For example, it is common for sub-Saharan countries to invite an international expert to coach or provide mental skills training in preparation for major games (e.g., Olympic games). It is therefore important for mental health professionals and clients to build rapport and understand cultural expectations and boundaries. Failure to meet basic cultural competencies may pose challenges to both the client and the practitioner. Research in Africa provides evidence that intersecting cultural compositions and norms including but not limited to, socialization, age, language, gender, religion, race, and sexual orientation (Hagan Jr. et al., 2019) play a pivotal role in the delivery of sport psychology services. For example, reports on elite athletes' mental health in South Africa (Muller, 2018) indicates that seeking sport psychology services is optional, and mental health practitioners are dubbed "head doctor." In an environment where there is stigma to seeking mental health care, it is paramount for the health care practitioner to have created the most conducive environment for athletes to seek help. The challenge noted in South Africa may not be isolated to South Africa. Other parts of the sub-Saharan countries may have similar experiences, particularly that it is not a requirement to see a psychologist in the region.

The authors of the present chapter have all had to deal with socio-cultural and spiritual issues in their practice. For example, a conflict and near fights between athletes in one of the national teams' camps led to the coaches and team management struggle to manage the situation. Following an investigation, the team leadership learnt that one of the athletes was accused of bewitching other athletes, his/her *muti* causing injuries and poor athletic performance to competitors within the team. This experience destabilized the camp and caused divisions in the team. It is therefore important for sport psychologists to be open minded and exercise caution. Labeling such experiences as paranoia can destabilize the team and lead to further divisions. The belief in such indigenous practice can be inconsistent with the psychologists' values and principles, but he or she has to mindful and respectful that they exist.

Interventions for mental health issues in sub-Saharan elite sport

Challenges that negatively impact diagnosis and treatment of mental ill-health in sub-Saharan Africa include the following: Stigmatization, poor provision, and limited supply of professionals, limited resources, and lack of regulation of the practice (Mbakile-Mahlanza et al., 2015). Clinical issues which impact diagnosis and treatment include, among other things, varied presentation of symptoms, different or unique perceived causes of mental ill-health, and a dearth of assessment and diagnostic tools which have been validated for African populations.

The most common mental health issues that we have observed among athletes in the region include major depressive disorder, anxiety and related disorders, post-traumatic stress disorder, substance use disorders and sleep disorders. Given the varied presentations seen in clinical practice, it is unlikely that any one theory, model or framework can address all of these difficulties and wedding them to a single approach will likely lead to poor clinical practice. Given that the purpose of treatment is to enable athletes to achieve optimum levels of mental well-being and performance, it is imperative for treatment to be athlete tailored. This resonates well with the idea of client response specificity in interpersonal psychotherapy.

In alleviating mental health issues among athletes, we ensure that our practices of counseling and psychotherapy are informed by both current scientific discoveries and the prevailing socio-cultural conditions. Generic treatments plans are unlikely to be successful without exploring specifically the issues relevant to the particular athletes. It is of paramount importance to consider athletes' circumstances in a careful and judicious manner in accordance with the practice of client response specificity. For example, in our experience, we have seen that social dimensions such as socio-economic status, family structure as well as educational levels can facilitate/trigger and/or diminish mental health problems.

How do Africans explain the occurrence of mental illnesses? Several studies have suggested varied causal attributions of mental illness in Africa. For example, Kinyua and Njagi (2013) found that Kenyans perceive mental illness to be caused by curses, misuse of drugs, and poor lifestyle. Opare-Henaku (2013) found that Ghanaians believe that among other things, causes of mental illness include spiritual forces. In Tanzania, Chikomo (2011) found that mental illnesses are not perceived as diseases but rather as the outcome of possession by evil spirits, witchcraft or curses. These attributions to mental illness have also been documented in Ethiopia by Teferra and Shibre (2012). Overall, the dominant causal attribution to mental illness in Africa is the supernatural elements. Mental health providers need to be cognizant of this because beliefs about causes on mental illness have been linked to help-seeking behaviors (Lynch & Medin, 2006). These beliefs also have implications for compliance with treatment.

A key element in good clinical practice is the use of empirically – supported treatment protocols. In this approach, interventions need to be empirically supported to be clinically effective and cost effective. In light of this, we believe that assessment tools used for diagnosis which have been imported from other cultures need to be modified based on assessment of their cultural appropriateness. Most tools for diagnosis and treatment of mental health issues have, however, been developed in Western countries and may not be useful or appropriate in non-western settings due to cultural and language differences. It is suggested then that when selecting scales or psychological tests, it is important to consider their relevance in relation to the athlete's cultural milieu. For example, in a commonly used tool for the diagnosis of depression, which has been developed in the Western world, one of the items reads "I am feeling blue." The respondent is asked to indicate the degree to which they are feeling blue and if they score high on this item, they are more likely to be classified with a degree of depression. Most people in sub-Saharan mental health practice are, however, unlikely to endorse this item due to a lack of understanding of what 'feeling blue' is in this context. Similarly, practitioners often rely on such other sources of information in a psychological or mental health assessment as records review, interviews, and behavioral observations. The types of protocols available and the considerations that went into producing them are culture-bound. Expectations of interview, ways of obtaining information through interview, considerations of confidentiality and disclosure are all culture-bound. The behaviors that an athlete will display in different settings and behavioral expectations are also culture-bound. All of these issues need to be taken into account when working with athletes. Practitioners desire as well as aim at performing psychological diagnoses that inform the choice of suitable clinical interventions to help athletes thrive and realize their rehabilitation goals. As a result, it is of utmost importance for psychologists to ensure that the tools that they use for diagnosis are appropriate. Unfortunately, we have very few tools that are appropriately translated and culturally sensitive to the specific context of sub- Saharan mental health diagnosis and treatment.

Treatment planning is a fundamental process and an effective treatment occurs as a multidisciplinary practice. Owing to this, clearly communicating clinical actions facilitates the provision of treatment as it creates a common frame of reference for collaborative practice. Further, it is important that mental health practitioners are able to justify their treatment decisions based on the available scientific evidence as well as in consideration of the patients' or athletes` cultural background and preferences. Pereira and colleagues (2017) emphasize integrating culture into rehabilitation to offer context specific suggestions for practice, which among others include beginning with the athlete and his or her family. This, on one hand, means taking into account their needs, what they hope to achieve, what is most important to them and their cultural background. For example, individual and group counseling interventions are employed in assisting the athletes to excel in their competitions while at the same time maintaining a stable mind. Athletes present varying issues informed by their cultural beliefs and customs, which affect their mental health. It is however worth noting that sub-Saharan athletes attend sessions with skepticism based on the fact that some have never been exposed to sport psychology services. This was specifically observed by one of the authors who worked with athletes during competitions; that some athletes attributed their poor performance to underlying psychosocial issues. Therefore, in addressing the problems, the psychologist settled for one on one intervention as opposed to team or group intervention.

Summary and recommendations

In summary, elite athletes' mental health issues in Africa are deeply related to cultural and religious beliefs and practices, and best tackled based on a very comprehensive, holistic assessment of the athlete, the athletes' strengths and limitations as well as the social and physical environment in which they live. It is incumbent upon practitioners to have deep knowledge of athletes` cultural customs, educational background, sport organizational cultures, as well as roles and expectations of sport federations.

In view of the mental health challenges experienced by elite athletes in sub-Saharan Africa, it is recommended that practitioners should:

- Demonstrate humility. The concept of Ubuntu is highly revered across the sub-Saharan region. It is important to be respectful, greet elders, and demonstrate kindness. Pomposity and self-importance is often interpreted as lack of respect.
- Demonstrate deep cultural competence (gender, age, language, religion, customs, and socialization). For example, minimize labeling behavior or client conduct even if it falls within conventional psychology concepts. The use of words such as paranoia can be

offensive to athletes. We recommend that issues be discussed within their context and the use of examples is key.

- Understand the different sport organizational cultures in sub-Saharan Africa. It is common that a government official with no knowledge either of sport or psychology can be appointed team manager or leader of the team. He or she may make decisions that affect athletes' mental readiness and in some cases, they may not be the most considerate. It is therefore important to exercise patience and put athletes' interest ahead of everyone in the team.
- Be informed of clients' educational background, mental skills knowledge, preferred language, and any other issue. Athletes may not understand or speak English and may also have different perspectives about sport psychology. Athletes may start off really quiet and it may take time for them to open up. It is important to fully understand them and exercise patience.
- Expose athletes to general life skills necessary for self and team management, because they need them beyond sport. This may be the only opportunity for them to learn life skills.
- Have full knowledge of mental health protocols, relevant issues, and requirements for that particular country. Failure to observe rules and national requirements can be interpreted as condescending and lack of respect.
- Allow for both individual and group sessions and respect athletes` differences. It is common for athletes to have different views and experiences informed by varying cultures, customs, and religions within the same team.
- Allow the athletes to make reference to their other personal issues as these may be contributing to their mental health. For example, it is common for athletes to make reference to their parents and grandparents use of indigenous herbs or rituals to address psychosocial issues.
- Deal with athletes independently without involving their coaches or team managers. Athletes may need someone other than their coach to share their experiences. For example, an athlete may need guidance and strength to inform his/her coach that he would like to move to a different coach. It is important to maintain confidentiality.
- Have follow-up sessions or supportive counseling for athletes. Athletes may not always initiate follow up sessions. It is important for the psychologist to be proactive.

References

Abu-Raddad, L. J., Ghanem, K. G., Feizzadeh, A., Setayesh, H., Calleja, J. M. G., & Riedner, G. (2013). HIV and other sexually transmitted infection research in the Middle East and North Africa: Promising progress? *Sexually Transmitted Infections 89*(Suppl 3), iii1–iii4. https://doi.org/10.1136/sextrans-2013-051373.

Ackah-Baidoo, P. (2016). Youth unemployment in resource-rich sub-Saharan Africa: A critical review. *The Extractive Industries and Society 3*(1), 249–261. https://doi.org/10.1016/j.exis.2015.11.010.

Adjaye, J. K. (2010). Reimagining sports: African athletes, defection, and ambiguous citizenship. *Africa Today 57*(2), 27–40.

Agbo, A. (2019, 23 August). Africa games: Fear in Rabat as Nigeria athletes threaten to boycott events. *Best Choice Sports*. https://bestchoicesports.com.ng/africa-games-fear-in-rabat-as-nigeria-athletes-threaten-to-boycott-events/

Akachi, Y., & Canning, D. (2007). The height of women in sub-Saharan Africa: The role of health, nutrition, and income in childhood. *Annals of Human Biology 34*(4), 397–410. https://doi.org/10.1080/03014460701452868

Alem, A., Desta, M., & Araya, M. (1995). Mental health in Ethiopia. *Ethiopian Journal of Health Development 9*, 47–62.

Amusa, L., & Toriola, A. L. (2010). The changing phases of physical education and sport in Africa: Can a uniquely African model emerge? *African Journal for Physical, Health Education, Recreation & Dance 16*(4), 666–680.

Baker, W. (1987). Political games: The meaning of international sport for independent Africa. In *Sport in Africa: Essays in social history* (pp. 272–295). Africana Publishing Company.

Chikomo, J. G. (2011). *Knowledge and attitudes of the Kinondoni community towards mental illness* (Doctoral dissertation, Stellenbosch: University of Stellenbosch).

Crick, L. (2010). Mental health in Africa: Findings from the Mental Health and Poverty Project. *International Review of Psychiatry 22*(6), 547–549. https://doi.org/10.3109/09540261.2010.535809.

Ford, P., Croix, M. D. S., Lloyd, R., Meyers, R., Moosavi, M., Oliver, J., Till, K., & Williams, C. (2011). The long-term athlete development model: Physiological evidence and application. *Journal of Sports Sciences 29*(4), 389–402. https://doi.org/10.1080/02640414.2010.536849.

France-Presse, A. (2016, August). Olympics: Three top Kenyan officials arrested. *GMA NewsOnline*. www.searchnewworld.com/search/search2.html?partid=rolbng&p=kenyan+olympic+official+arrested&subid=004.

Gureje, O., & Alem, A. (2000). Mental health policy development in Africa. *Bulletin of the World Health Organization 78*(4), 475–482.

Hagan Jr., J. E., & Schack, T. (2017). The influence of indigenous culture on sport psychology practice: Challenges and prospects. *Psychology and Behavioral Science International Journal* 7(4). https://pub.uni-bielefeld.de/record/2916070.

Hagan Jr., J. E., Schack, T., & Schinke, R. (2019). Sport psychology practice in Africa: Do culture-specific religion and spirituality matter? *Advances in Social Sciences Research Journal 6*(3). https://pub.uni-bielefeld.de/record/2934574

Hernández, A., Ruano, A. L., Marchal, B., San Sebastián, M., & Flores, W. (2017). Engaging with complexity to improve the health of indigenous people: A call for the use of systems thinking to tackle health inequity. *International Journal for Equity in Health 16*(1), 26. https://doi.org/10.1186/s12939-017-0521-2.

Ikulayo, P. B., & Semidara, J. A. (2011). Culturally informed sport psychology practice: Nigeriain perspective. *Journal of Clinical Sport Psychology 5*(4), 339–349. https://doi.org/10.1123/jcsp.5.4.339.

Kinyua, B., & Njagi, E. (2013). *Knowledge and perceptions about mental illnesses among Kenyan immigrants living in Jyvaskyla, Finland* [Fi=AMK-opinnäytetyö|sv=YH-examensarbete|en=Bachelor's thesis|, Jamk University of Applied Sciences]. www.theseus.fi/handle/10024/65469.

Lin, J. (2012) Youth bulge: A demographic dividend or a demographic bomb in developing countries? World Bank, http://blogs.worldbank.org/developmenttalk/youth-bulge-a- demographic-dividend-or-a-demographic-bomb-in-developing-countries (accessed 20 January 2014).

Lynch, E., & Medin, D. (2006). Explanatory models of illness: A study of within-culture variation. *Cognitive Psychology 53*(4), 285–309.

Mbakile-Mahlanza, L., Manderson, L., & Ponsford, J. (2015). The experience of traumatic brain injury in Botswana. *Neuropsychological Rehabilitation 25*(6), 936–958.

Muller, A. (2018). After the whistle: How do elite athletes deal with the injuries nobody can see? *Daily Maverick*. www.searchnewworld.com/search/search2.html?partid=rolbng&p=athletes+mental+health+south+africa&subid=004

Novitsky, V., Prague, M., Moyo, S., Gaolathe, T., Mmalane, M., Yankinda, E. K., Chakalisa, U., Lebelonyane, R., Khan, N., Powis, K. M., Widenfelt, E., Gaseitsiwe, S., Dryden-Peterson, S. L., Holme, M. P., De Gruttola, V., Bachanas, P., Makhema, J., Lockman, S., & Essex, M. (2018). High HIV-1 RNA among newly diagnosed people in Botswana. *AIDS Research and Human Retroviruses 34*(3), 300–306. https://doi.org/10.1089/aid.2017.0214.

Opare-Henaku, A. (2013). *Notions of spirits as agents of mental illness among the Akan of Ghana: A cultural-psychological exploration*. Virginia Commonwealth University.

Peart, H. (2005, August 3). *Kenya plea over athlete defection*. http://news.bbc.co.uk/2/hi/africa/4740385.stm.

Pereira, A., Fish, J., Malley, D., & Bateman, A. (2017). The importance of culture in holistic neuropsychological rehabilitation: Suggestions for improving cultural competence. In *Neuropsychological rehabilitation: The International Handbook* (pp. 530–534). Taylor & Francis.

Selamu, M., Asher, L., Hanlon, C., Medhin, G., Hailemariam, M., Patel, V., Thornicroft, G., & Fekadu, A. (2015). Beyond the biomedical: Community resources for mental health care in rural Ethiopia. *PloS One 10*(5), e0126666. https://doi.org/10.1371/journal.pone.0126666.

Serpa, S., & Stambulova, N. (2016). Bola Ikulayo (1948–2016). *International Journal of Sport and Exercise Psychology 14*(2), 188–193. https://doi.org/10.1080/1612197X.2016.1180748.

Teferra, S., & Shibre, T. (2012). Perceived causes of severe mental disturbance and preferred interventions by the Borana semi-nomadic population in southern Ethiopia: A qualitative study. *BMC Psychiatry 12*(1), 79.

Tshube, T., & Hanrahan, S. J. (2016). Sport psychology in Botswana: A prime breeding ground. *International Journal of Sport and Exercise Psychology 14*(2), 126–134. https://doi.org/10.1080/1612197X.2016.1142462.

4

MENTAL HEALTH IN BRAZILIAN SPORT

Olympic, Paralympic, and soccer athletes

Franco Noce, Varley Teoldo da Costa, Marcelo Callegari Zanetti, Maria Regina Ferreira Brandão, Ciro Winckler, Fabrízio Veloso Rodrigues, Aline Arias Wolff, and Cristina Carvalho de Melo

Introduction

Brazil is a country of continental proportions, with the fifth largest population in the world originally made up of different ethnic groups, such as indigenous (natives), Portuguese (main colonizers), and Africans (brought to Brazil as slaves at the time of colonization). From a cultural perspective, the important contribution of immigrants (European, Japanese, and Arabic) to Brazilian traditions (Brandão and Vieira, 2013) is highlighted. From the economic view point, the recent reforms have improved the stability of the economy, but the country still struggles with high levels of social inequality, which require a government agenda that prioritizes their confrontation, aiming at a more just and civilized society (Paiva et al., 2016). From the perspective of education, the Federal Constitution states that "education" is "a right for all, and a duty of the State and the family." Nevertheless, in 2013, the results of the Brazilian Institute of Geography and Statistics point to 8.3% of illiteracy in the country (Lacruz et al., 2019).

The Brazilian public health system, entitled "Unique Health System – SUS," was instituted in 1988. Since then, the Brazilian population has the right to universal and free health care, financed with resources from the Union, State, Federal District, and Municipalities (Paim, 2018). As an integral part of the SUS, the Brazilian mental health care system was established in the country in the 1990s. Sharing the same principles of SUS, it is a public system, with a municipal, community, and articulated basis, focused on mental health care. These systems are composed of Centers of Psychosocial Attention (CAPS); Centers of Coexistence; Residential Therapeutic Services (SRT); Mental Health Ambulatories; and General Hospitals. The Municipal, State, and National Health Councils and the Mental Health Conferences ensure the participation and protagonism of mental health users and their families in the management of the SUS, as well as in the construction of the Mental Health care system (BRAZIL, 2005). It is important to highlight that around 30 years after its implementation, SUS is a system that still faces big challenges (Paim, 2018). Recently, however, Brazil has been experiencing a perceptible reduction in poverty and income inequality, with an improvement in access to health, education, and assistance services for the most vulnerable population.

Sport Psychology in Brazil

The first records of psychology's performance in sport date back to 1954 (João Carvalhaes with soccer referees), even preceding the regulation of the profession of psychologist in the country, which occurred in 1962. Currently in Brazil there are two national associations of sports psychology and several regional associations that have as primary objectives the organization and dissemination of the "new science" and the development of scientific studies (Noce et al., 2016). Evidence points to a growth of scientific production within the area of Sport Psychology in Brazil over the years (Vieira et al., 2019).

Sports mental health in Brazil, general considerations

To arrive at contextualized understanding of mental health, it is important to take into consideration the Brazilian reality, particularly the impact of social and economic determinants on mental health in Brazil (DSS). The DSS are the social, economic, cultural, ethnic, psychological, and behavioral factors that influence the occurrence of health problems and their risk factors in the population (Buss & Pellegrini Filho, 2007).

Economic and social conditions have an important effect on the health-disease relationship. According to Buss et al. (2016) socioeconomic differences in a society causes increased vulnerability in certain groups. From a "physical-material aspects" perspective, income differences influence health due to the scarcity of resources of individuals and the absence of investments in community infrastructure (education, transport, sanitation, housing, health services). From a "psychosocial factors" perspective, the perception and experience of people in unequal societies cause stress and harm to health (Buss & Pellegrini Filho, 2007). Specifically for Brazil, it has been possible to note a marked imbalance between the regions for decades, for example the huge difference between the riches of some large southeastern cities and the poverty of a northeastern Brazilian favela (Richeport, 1984). The Dahlgren & Whitehead model (1991) presents the DSS arranged in layers ranging from individual determinants (related to personal characteristics, behavior, and lifestyle) to socioeconomic policies (aimed at sustainable development reducing social and economic inequalities). The more the determinants move away from the core (behavioral factors), the less control a society has over conditions, increasing vulnerability to mental health impacts (Figure 4.1).

In the competitive sports context, a large number of athletes are strongly impacted by several socioeconomic determinants. For example, in many sport teams, especially in the youth academy, it is not difficult to find athletes who face basic difficulties in adequate nutrition (necessary to meet the energy demands for a competitive sports practice). Normally, conditions of sanitation and access to health are also precarious in some families. This ends up predisposing the young athlete to vulnerable conditions, increasing the risk of injuries and illnesses. In the following we will comment on the organization of the main sports institutions in Brazil and how the health sector, especially sports psychology, operates to support the athletes.

Organization of the institutions of competitive sport in Brazil

The main sports institutions in Brazil are the Brazilian Olympic Committee (COB), the Brazilian Paralympic Committee (CPB) and the Brazilian Soccer Confederation (CBF).

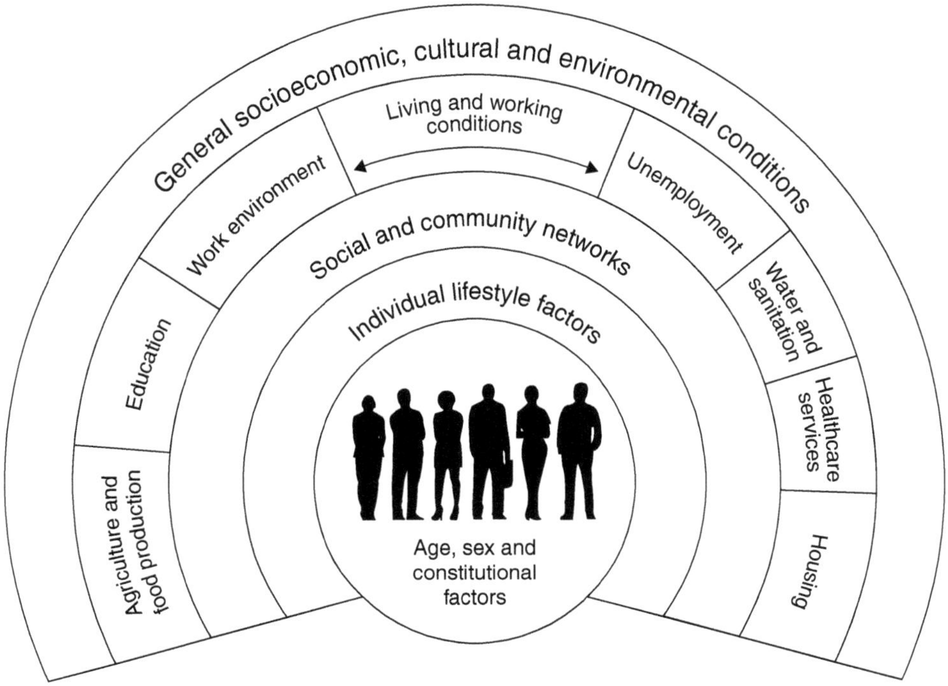

FIGURE 4.1 Social determinants: Dahlgren & Whitehead's model
Source: Dahlgren & Whitehead, 1991

Further, there are 30 confederations for Olympic and 23 for non-Olympic sports. Next we will understand, in a synthetic way, the organization and a little bit of the past, present, and future of these institutions.

Brazilian Olympic Committee

The Brazilian Olympic Committee (COB) is a non-governmental organization, affiliated to the International Olympic Committee (IOC), which works in the technical, administrative and political management of national sport. The COB's mission is to develop and represent with excellence the high performance sport of Brazil. COB strives for international top-level representation in the main world competitions by improving the sports results of the Brazil Team. They further strive to promote the system by raising raise the management maturity of the COB and its 35 affiliated confederations and strengthening the image of Brazilian Olympic sport.

Regarding the mental preparation service, in a not too distant past, the relationship between psychology and sport was only considered when analyzing a poor performance or defeat. The figure of the psychologist was considered a novelty and this kind of work was valued only when something was not going well. For several Olympic cycles, the mental preparation area was gradually implemented with the participation of few professionals, often working in isolation and certainly not enough to meet the high demand. The Beijing Games, in 2008, were a milestone for calling attention to the need to include psychological preparation in the athletes' training routine in a systematic manner.

From the end of 2014, the Brazilian Olympic Committee decided to invest even more in the systematization of psychological preparation work and brought together some professionals who were already operating with Olympic athletes in a working group. The area was then named Mental Preparation. After the 2016 Games, the area became part of the Olympic Laboratory (LO). Therefore, another important step in the consolidation of the area was taken, since in addition to maintaining the attention and intervention with athletes and coaches, the area also began to dedicate itself to the production of scientific knowledge, emphasizing even more, its practices on evidence.

Currently, psychological preparation is considered a fundamental part of an athlete's preparation, along with the technical/tactical and physical part. We can state that the main reason for this change is the successful work that Brazilian psychologists have been doing in recent years (Hallage, Wolff, & Dutra, 2017). COB has two contracted mental preparation professionals, a psychologist, a coach, and nine psychologists serve the institution as external collaborators.

Recently the mental preparation area has been expanded to include a focus on mental health. This was already an old desire, due to the large number of athletes with clinical and subclinical demands and in psychic suffering, and since the publication of the IOC consensus on mental health (Reardon et al., 2019), the initiative has gained more space within the institution. The search for mental health assistance among athletes is still seen as taboo, and psychopathology is still stigmatized in sports culture (Bauman, 2016), also in Brazil. Fortunately, in recent years, large institutions and athletes around the world are making this important issue known, which deserves to be highlighted because it positively influences all sports organizations and encourages programs to be addressed to improve the conditions of support and prevention in mental health. In Brazil we have seen this in the form of many outstanding athletes (Olympic level) who faced great difficulties and frustrations who had the courage to speak openly about their problems and their search for help from mental health professionals to overcome these adversities. This movement has gained momentum and attracted media attention. The promotion of these cases encouraged other athletes to seek help and sensitized institutions to implement the mental health service for athletes.

Brazilian Paralympic Committee

The Brazilian Paralympic Committee was created in 1995 and today serves as the entity that governs the adapted sport in Brazil. It represents and leads the Paralympic movement in the country and seeks the promotion and development of high performance sports for people with disabilities. It is based in the Paralympic Training Center located in the city of São Paulo, a facility with 95,000 square meters of constructed area and that can be used for training, competitions and exchanges of athletes and teams from 15 Paralympic disciplines. Differently from the Olympic Committee, the Paralympic Committee has a mixed management model, besides the international representativeness it works as a confederation of four sports modalities, athletics, swimming, weightlifting, and sport shooting.

In 1996, the managers of the Paralympic Committee understood that the sport would only evolve if it made a partnership with science. A multidisciplinary team was then formed in which the Sport Psychology was inserted. Until the 2008 cycle, the work was developed in a format with the Sport Psychology team attending all the Paralympic modalities in punctual conditions and in the periods in which the athletes were called to train and/or compete. In the preparation for the London Paralympic games there was a change of attendance, the multiprofessional teams started to focus on the specialized attendance in the modalities. Therefore, psychology professionals were able to direct their knowledge specialization to only one modality. Athletics and swimming were modalities that included these professionals in their technical committee that went to the 2012 games. The Rio Paralympic Games in 2016 became a milestone for the Sport Psychology in the CPB, mainly due to the results achieved during the Paralympic Games, the Sport Psychology was endorsed as an important part of the athletes' preparation program and started to count on the participation of different professionals in the area as members of the CPB staff and composing a team of professionals that would fulfill the demands of the national teams

The psychology team of the Brazilian Paralympic Committee adopts, as its main guiding action, the implementation of a high performance program for Paralympic athletes in order to develop and apply performance-oriented mental training methods (Samulski, Noce, & Costa, 2011). All actions are based on psychophysiological precepts and monitored with the help of technological tools, using the maintenance and promotion of quality of life. In other words, mental preparation of the athlete is advocated as a key to develop skills and strategies needed for high level sport performance. When it comes to athlete mental health, the picture is less impressive. Actually, the Brazilian Paralympic committee currently has no mental health sector in their organizational structure and no systematic services implemented.

Brazilian Soccer Confederation

Soccer in Brazil is huge. Brazil has 7020 soccer clubs registered with the confederation, from which 1430 clubs are active and fully functioning and 874 clubs are soccer professionals (Ernst & Young, 2019). Due to the sheer size of the federation, one would imagine that the professional soccer clubs in Brazil have well established cross-disciplinary support teams to meet the technical, tactical, physical, and psychological demands in the formation process of young athletes, including the services needed to support the footballers' mental health and performance. However, this is not the reality. A recent survey showed that of the 20 professional clubs in the first division of Brazilian league in 2020, only four clubs have the figure of the psychologist acting directly with the professional team and only one club reports a having a professional in the area of performance psychology depicted in the organization chart of its professional soccer department (Costa, 2020). In women's professional soccer (first division) the presence of a sports psychologist hardly exists.

The presence of the clinical psychologist is observed in the youth male categories according to the requirements imposed by the Pelé Law (Law 9615/98). In order to obtain the official license as a certified talent development club (CCF), issued by CBF, clubs need to prove that they offer psychological assistance through a professional registered with the Federal Council of Psychology. The mandatory presence of the psychologist in the youth categories was an achievement to all those engaged in soccer. Still, the working conditions are quite precarious. The majority of clubs have only one professional responsible for five to seven different categories of athletes, with approximately 30 athletes in each category. This generates a situation of extreme difficulty in the maintenance of the individual attendance and work of quality. A reason for this is that a psychologist attends on average 210 athletes, and furthermore meets demands and requests that arise from coaches and directors. From the organizational point of view, the psychologist in soccer clubs (when it exists) is inserted in the medical department (together with the doctor, physiotherapist, and nutritionist). This scenario occurs in the national youth and professional teams, being requested to join the technical committee upon demand.

In soccer, mental health problems are known to affect male and female athletes with success and failure (Ladwig, Kunrath, Luckaschek, et al., 2012) at the beginning of their careers (Blakelock, Chen, & Prescott, 2016), and in the process of transitioning from a sports career (Park, Lavallee, & Tod, 2013). In other words, it is noteworthy that in all sports stages of a soccer athlete's sporting life, problems related to mental health are present and can lead to serious and lethal situations (Ladwig, Kunrath, Luckaschek et al., 2012).

Evidence suggests that some groups are more vulnerable and susceptible to mental health problems in soccer. These groups are constituted by athletes with injury problems (Cezarino, Grüninger, & Silva, 2020), overtraining and demotivation (Fagundes, Noce, Albuquerque, et al., 2019), depression and anxiety (Pujals & Vieira, 2008), burnout and perfectionism symptoms (Bicalho & Costa, 2018).

It is observed that a large portion of Brazilian soccer athletes have a certain resistance and negligence, ignorance and prejudice regarding the need to seek psychological support inside or outside the club to deal with mental health problems. This problem has also been reported in the literature with soccer athletes of other nationalities, especially males (Wood, Harrison, & Kucharska, 2017). It is noteworthy that in Brazil, considered the country of football and five-time world champion, it appears that both on the part of the confederation, federation, and the clubs themselves there is no institutional policy to take care of the mental health of athletes. Existing shares can be classified as isolated shares or inserted only in the base categories. In this sense, making an analysis of the concern with the mental health of the Brazilian soccer player without understanding the complex ways in which the sport is seen and treated in Brazil could lead to misconceptions and irrelevant findings. Our football-art in the value system that permeates Brazilian sport was polished in a positive valuation of the football player as having an innate, rare, singular, specific, and exclusive characteristic, in other words, Brazilian players would play well because they would be gifted with supposedly intrinsic natural qualities, such as individual talent and natural genius, which would be expressed by their skill, malice, and spontaneity (Brandão & Vieira, 2013). However, this facet of innate talent positively valued by our "football culture" brings as a consequence a player who has little emotional preparation during his career as is true of the institutions that work with him. From this observation, it is clear that the great challenge for Brazilian football is to change the belief that the player's pure, genuine, innate, irreverent, playful talent, does not need effort to be improved and does not need specialized psychological work.

The status of mental health service provision in Brazil: An investigation

One question, answered above, is how many people are working in the Sport Psychology and mental health area? The answer was that it was clearly not enough. Another question is how do the people who are in the field approach their work? When we set out to write this chapter, we quickly realized that there was no overview of how mental health services were organized and used in Brazil. Therefore we decided to look into the matters ourselves. To do so, we sent out an interview script (through Google Forms) to 104 Brazilian sport psychologists and other professionals who work with the mental health of athletes involved in competition (61.5% female and 38.5% male, with psychology education (76%) and specific education in sports psychology (53%) distributed to include people working in several sport institutions and across the country, see Table 4.1). Questions around mental health in competitive athletes

TABLE 4.1 Sociodemographic characteristics of participants

Characteristic	*n*	%
Gender		
Male	40	38.5
Female	64	61.5
Academic graduation		
Psychology	79	76
Physical education	13	12.5
Psychology and Physical Education	11	10.6
Physical Education and Pedagogy	1	0.9
Specialization in Sport Psychology		
Yes	55	53
No	49	47
Master's degree		
Yes	55	53
No	49	47
Ph.D.		
Yes	28	27
No	76	73
Field of action		
Athletes and teams	85	82
Athletes	16	15.2
Teams	3	2.8
Work contract		
Self-employed	72	69
Hired by the company	32	31
Who is the contractor		
Team / Club / Institution	78	75
Athlete	26	25
Practice field in Sport Psychology[a]		
Practical field work	87	83.7
Attendance of athletes in office	64	61.5
Scientific research	46	44.2
Teaching	44	42.3
Consultancy	37	35.6
Supervision of other professionals	47	45.2
Supervising students	49	47.1
Main sports practice area		
Olympic sport	46	44.2
Paralympic sport	7	6.7
Amateur sports (also includes social projects)	31	29.8
Soccer	20	19.2

Note. N = 104. Participants were on average 41.2 years old (SD = 10.4), and length of experience as a Sports Psychologist from 10.8 years (SD = 8.8).

[a] The sum of the characteristic Practice field in Sport Psychology is greater than 100% because many professionals reported having more than 1 field of activity.

in Brazil were based on recent consensus statements about mental health of athletes elaborated by the International Society of Sport Psychology (Schinke et al., 2017; Henriksen et al., 2019; Henriksen et al., 2020) and the European Federation of Sport Psychology (Moesch et al., 2018). Questions revolved around (1) monitoring of emotions and behaviors, (2) intervention strategies, (3) clinical psychology/psychiatry indication, (4) barriers to working with mental health, (5) concern of the institution with mental health, (6) institutional program for mental health prevention, (7) coaches' concern with emotional health, and (8) suggestions to improve work around athlete mental health. The script included questionnaire like questions as well as qualitative questions that allowed insights into the strategies adopted by different Sport Psychology professionals, their respective institutions and coaches, as well as work proposals and encountered barriers.

Regarding the "Monitoring of emotions and behaviors" the practitioners highlighted strategies such as: direct observation and participation in training and competitions, use of psychometric instruments as self-filling questionnaires (e.g., mood states, anxiety, and recovery), conducting interviews, group dynamics, online monitoring (through WhatsApp), self report, use of neuro and biofeedback, individual care, conversations with family, use of training diaries, meetings with the multidisciplinary team, Eletroencephalogram (EEG) monitoring, coach statements, physiological indicators, and complaints by athletes.

In terms of "Intervention strategies – emotions and behaviours," the practitioners mentioned: supportive actions, psychoeducation programs, individualized care, group dynamics, self-knowledge promotion, breathing techniques, relaxation, visualization, mentalization, meditation, concentration, attention, biofeedback use, positive reinforcement, hypnosis, awareness, periodic conversations with the technical team and athletes, positive internal dialogue, education and emotional regulation, setting goals and objectives, developing coping strategies, mindfulness, cognitive-behavioral techniques, compassion, cognitive stress control, psychological skills training, imaginary training, and transcranial stimulation.

In the "Clinical Psychology/Psychiatry Indication" category, it was demonstrated that 62.5% of the participants have already indicated the work of Clinical Psychology and/or Psychiatry, citing different reasons: There was psychological abuse by the staff toward the athlete, the athlete presented disorders such as anorexia, anxiety, depression, visual delirium, self-mutilation, bipolar disorder, obsessive compulsive disorder, panic attacks, family and personal problems, need for medication and deeper diagnosis, suicidal thoughts.

As "Barriers to working with mental health" were mentioned: lack of acceptance by the athlete and the family, lack of self-knowledge, lack of team planning and time, low credibility of Sport Psychology among the technical team, misinformation, lack of support and resistance by coaches and supervisors, lack of structure and investment, multiple athletes' trips, lack of priorities, preconception of some managers, athletes and teams, family issues, excessive demand from the coach, fear of the athlete to expose his weaknesses and lack of work synchrony of coaches and athletes.

68% of the practitioners experienced that their institution was "Concerned with mental health." They mentioned the adoption of some measures by their institutions, such as inclusion of the sports psychologist in the trainings and competitions, daily monitoring of the athletes' mental health status, presence of social assistant, possibility of external referrals (Psychiatrists and Clinical Psychologists), systematic monitoring of the sports performance decline, availability of psychology professionals in all categories and search for a multidisciplinary work involving psychologists and different professionals of the technical commission.

However, only 38.5% of practitioners stated that they had an "Institutional program of mental health prevention." The ones that did cited the accomplishment of: lectures and meetings on the subject with other professionals and diverse contents, conversations with the family, orientation with the athletes, psychological evaluation, group dynamics, programs of prevention of mental health problems, weekly accompaniment with multidisciplinary team, study groups, and that in some institutions there are no special programs directed to this purpose.

82% of practitioners said their coaches were "concerned with the emotional health" of their athletes. This was evidenced by the coaches believing in and understand the importance of the Sport Psychologist's work, performing monitoring of the team's and/or athletes' performance, behavior, and difficulties, seeking individualization of the work with each athlete based on the profile identified by the sport psychologist, and establishing contact and systematic support to the athlete when identifying the need.

The practioners provided several "suggestions to improved mental health services." These included: To follow possible mental suffering scenarios of athletes, to develop work since the sport initiation, to expand the qualification of the professionals involved with the subject, to seek assistance from the public power, autonomous professionals and universities, basic knowledge of Sport Psychology by the technical commission, to create environments and training courses that promote greater mental health in athletes, to elaborate strategies to face disorders, to include the family of athletes in mental health programs, to create events on Sport Psychology, mandatory presence of the Mental Health Professional in the sports environments, clinical training of the sports psychologist with action based on solid evidence, implementation of mental health programs in the training routine (not only with the aim of performance) greater dialogue between professionals in the field for the development of protocols and mental preparation programs, creation of lectures and workshops, sensitization of sports managers about the importance of developing mental health programs, having a mental health sector with psychologists and psychiatrists.

Considerations

Brazil being a country with so many socioeconomic challenges and taking into consideration the impacts that these determinants have on mental health, it is possible to see the extent to which competitive sport in the country can be affected. Several institutional measures can be implemented in order to minimize the impacts on mental health of athletes, coaches, and other professionals inserted in this environment.

In all the Brazilian institutions investigated, it could be seen that there is still a strong association of the sport psychologist's activity with the clinical and not the performance component. Although the clinical and health component is something fundamental, this aspect limits the insertion of the professional in Olympic and Paralympic teams and in professional soccer. A recommendation would be to provide information to sports managers on the difference of roles between health and performance, even though in many cases the professional can perform both functions. The mental preparation field, of the different institutions that compose the Brazilian sport organism, shows that both COB and CPB believe that the mental health work of the athletes may bring significant results in the improvement of their mental health, in the adequate notification of psychopathological diagnoses and consequently in the conduction of effective treatments. Therefore, it is expected that the culture of Olympic and

Paralympic sport will become more supportive of alleviating psychic suffering and thereby more conducive to mental health and consequently, more conducive to the best performances.

In Brazilian soccer, it has been found that the confederation (CBF), the federation and the clubs themselves do not have an institutional policy to provide mental health care for athletes. The existing actions can be classified as isolated actions or inserted only in the youth categories.

Advances are needed in soccer to change the current Brazilian reality. Thus, it is necessary to develop educational campaigns that have the purpose of disseminating and informing managers, coaches, members of the technical staff, and especially the athletes about the importance and need to care for their mental health.

In order to be more efficient, these campaigns need the institutional support of the Fédération Internationale de Football Association (FIFA), the main continental confederations such as the South American Soccer Confederation (CONMEBOL) and the Union of European Football Associations (UEFA) and entities such as ISSP (International Society of Sport Psychology), South American Net of Sport Psychology (Red PsySur). In summary, because Brazil is an open country and Brazilian sport coaches and managers listen to world experts, we really would benefit from a worldwide movement made by renowned entities, athletes, coaches, psychologists, and other professionals involved in high performance sport. This movement would have a single purpose to improve the quality of mental health of all those involved in the sport. Finally, especially athletes need to be aware that their mental health is a variable that should be non-negotiable, since not only the athlete's performance but also other segments of his or her life depend greatly on it. Athletes who have a good mental health level are more likely to achieve their sports goals as well as being physically, psychologically, and socially healthier people. For these athletes, "Nothing is more important than their own mental health."

References

Alhojailan, M. I. (2012). Thematic analysis: A critical review of its process and evaluation. *West East Journal of Social Sciences 1*(1), 39–47. https://fac.ksu.edu.sa/sites/default/files/ta_thematic_analysis_dr_mohammed_alhojailan.pdf.

Bauman, N. J. (2016). The stigma of mental health in athletes: Are mental toughness and mental health seen as contradictory in elite sport? *British Journal of Sports Medicine 50*(3), 135–136. http://dx.doi.org/10.1136/bjsports-2015–095570.

Bicalho, C. C. F., & Costa, V. T. (2018). Burnout in elite athletes: A systematic review. *Cuadernos de Psicologia del Deporte 18*(1), 89–102. http://hdl.handle.net/10201/56104.

Blakelock, D. J., Chen, M. A., & Prescott, T. (2016). Psychological distress in elite adolescent soccer players following deselection. *Journal of Clinical Sport Psychology 10*(1), 59–77. https://doi.org/10.1123/jcsp.2015-0010.

Brandão, M. R. F., & Vieira, L. F. (2013). Athletes' careers in Brazil: Research and application in the land of ginga. In N. Stambulova, & T. V. Ryba (Eds.), *Athletes' careers across cultures* (pp. 63–72). Routledge.

Brasil. (2005). Reforma psiquiátrica e política de saúde mental no Brasil [Psychiatric reform and mental health policy in Brazil]. Ministério da Saúde, Secretaria deAtenção à Saúde. https://bvsms.saude.gov.br/bvs/publicacoes/Relatorio15_anos_Caracas.pdf.

Buss, P. M., & Pellegrini Filho, A. (2007). A saúde e seus determinantes sociais [Health and its social determinants]. *Physis revista saúde coletiva 17*(1), 77–93. http://dx.doi.org/10.1590/S0103-73312007000100006.

Buss, P. M., Chamas, C., Faid, M., & Morel, C. (2016). Desenvolvimento, saúde e política internacional: a dimensão da pesquisa & inovação [Development, health, and international policy: The research and innovation dimension]. *Cadernos desaúde pública 32*(s2), s1–s12. http://dx.doi.org/10.1590/0103-311X00046815.

Cezarino, L. G., Grüninger, B. L. S., & Silva, R. S. (2020). Injury profile in a Brazilian first-division youth soccer team: A prospective study. *Journal of Athletic Training 55*(3), 295–302. http://doi.org/10.4085/1062-6050-449-18.

Costa, V. T. (2020). *Levantamento do serviço de Psicologia do Esporte e Coaching Esportivo em clubes da série A do futebol Brasileiro: Ano base 2020* [Survey of the Sport Psychology and Sports Coaching service in Brazilian football series A clubs: Base year 2020]. www.lapes.com.br/lapes/index.php/publicacoes#

Dahlgren, G., & Whitehead, M. (1991). *Policies and Strategies to Promote Social Equity in Health.* Institute for Futures Studies. www.ncbi.nlm.nih.gov/books/NBK221240/.

Ernst & Young. (2019). Impacto do Futebol Brasileiro [Impact of Brazilian Football]. Confederação Brasileira de Futebol. https://conteudo.cbf.com.br/cdn/201912/20191213172843_346.pdf.

Fagundes, L. H. S., Noce, F., Albuquerque, M. R., Andrade, A. G. P., & Teoldo da Costa, V. (2019). Can motivation and overtraining predict burnout in professional soccer athletes in different periods of the season?. *International Journal of Sport and Exercise Psychology.* https://doi.org/10.1080/1612197X.2019.1655778.

Faleiros, F., Käppler, C., Pontes, F. A. R., Silva, S. S. D. C., Goes, F. D. S. N. D., & Cucick, C. D. (2016). Use of virtual questionnaire and dissemination as a data collection strategy in scientific studies. *Texto & Contexto-Enfermagem 25*(4). http://dx.doi.org/10.1590/0104-07072016003880014

Fletcher, A. J. (2017). Applying critical realism in qualitative research: Methodology meets method. *International Journal of Social Research Methodology 20*(2), 181–194. http://doi.org/10.1080/13645579.2016.1144401.

Hallage, S., Wolff, A. A., & Dutra, A. (2017). Psicologia do esporte e o legado olímpico [Sport psychology and the Olympic legacy]. In C. Medeiros, & A. Lacerda (Org.), *Psicologia e esporte na atualidade: reflexões necessárias* (pp. 19–29). Pasavento.

Henriksen, K., Schinke, R., Moesch, K., McCann, S., Parham, W. D., Larsen, C. H., & Terry, P. (2019). Consensus statement on improving the mental health of high performance athletes. *International Journal of Sport and Exercise Psychology.* http://doi.org/10.1080/1612197X.2019.1570473.

Henriksen, K., Schinke, R., McCann, S., Durand-Bush, N., Moesch, K., Parham, W. D., Larsen, C. H., Cogan, K., Donaldsen, A., Poczwardowski, A., Noce F., & Hunziker, J. (2020). Athlete mental health in the Olympic/ Paralympic quadrennium: A multi-societal consensus statement. *International Journal of Sport and Exercise Psychology.* https://doi.org/10.1080/1612197X.2020.1746379.

Lacruz, A. J., Américo, B. L., & Carniel, F. (2019). Indicadores de qualidade na educação: análise discriminante dos desempenhos na Prova Brasil [Quality indicators in education: Discriminant analysis of the performances in ProvaBrasil]. *Revista Brasileira de Educação 24.* https://doi.org/10.1590/s1413-24782019240002

Ladwig, K. H., Kunrath, S., Luckaschek, K., & Baumert, J. (2012). The railway suicide death of a famous German football player: Impact on the subsequent frequency of railway suicide acts in Germany. *Journal of Affective Disorders 136*(1–2), 194–198. https://doi.org/10.1016/j.jad.2011.09.044.

Moesch, K., Kenttä, G., Kleinert, J., Quignon-Fleuret, C., Cecil, S., & Bertollo, M. (2018). FEPSAC position statement: Mental health disorders in elite athletes and models of service provision. *Psychology of Sport and Exercise 38*, 61–71. https://doi.org/10.1016/j.psychsport.2018.05.013.

Noce, F., Vieira, L. F., & Costa, V. (2016). Brazil. In R. J. Schinke, K. R. McGannom, & B. Smith (Eds.), *Routledge International Handbook of Sport Psychology* (pp. 56–64). Routledge.

NVivo. (2020). NVivo qualitative data analysis software. In (Release 1.0 ed.): QSR International Pty Ltd, Melbourne, Australia.

Paim, J. S. (2018). Sistema Único de Saúde (SUS) aos 30 anos. [Thirty years of the Unified Health System (SUS)]. *Ciência & Saúde Coletiva 23*(6), 1723–1728. https://doi.org/10.1590/1413-81232018236.09172018.

Paiva, A. B., Mesquita, A. C. S., Jaccoud, L., & Passos, L. (2016). *O novo regime fiscal e suas implicações para a política de assistência social no Brasil* [The new tax regime and its implications for social assistance policy in Brazil]. Instituto de Pesquisa Econômica Aplicada. http://repositorio.ipea.gov.br/bitstream/11058/7267/1/NT_n27_Disoc.pdf.

Park, S., Lavallee, D., & Tod, D. (2013). Athletes' career transition out of sport: A systematic review. *International Review of Sport and Exercise Psychology 6*(1), 22–53. https://doi.org/10.1080/1750984X.2012.687053.

Pujals, C., & Vieira, L. F. (2008). Análise dos fatores psicológicos que interferem no comportamento dos atletas de futebol de campo [Analysis of psychological factors which interfere in soccer athletes' behaviour]. *Journal of Physical Education 13*(1), 89–97. www.periodicos.uem.br/ojs/index.php/RevEducFis/article/view/3756

Reardon, C. L., Hainline, B., Aron, C. M., Baron, D., Baum, A. L., Bindra, A., Budgett, R., Campriani, N., Castaldelli-Maia, J. M., Currie, A., Derevensky, J. L., Glick, I. D., Gorczynski, P., Gouttebarge, V., Grandner, M. A., Han, D. H., McDuff, D., Mountjoy, M., Polat, A., … Engebretsen, L. (2019). Mental health in elite athletes: International Olympic Committee consensus statement. *British Journal of Sports Medicine 53*(11), 667–699. http://doi.org/10.1136/bjsports-2019-100715.

Richeport, M. (1984). Strategies and outcomes of introducing a mental health plan in Brazil. *Social Science & Medicine 19*(3), 261–271. https://doi.org/10.1016/0277-9536(84)90217-X.

Samulski, D., Noce, F., & Costa, V. (2011). Mental preparation. In: Y. C. Vanlandewijck, & W. R. Thompson (Ed.), *The Paralympic Athlete* (pp.198–213). Wiley-Blackwell.

Schinke, R. J., Stambulova, N. B., Si, G., & Moore, Z. (2017). International Society of Sport Psychology position stand: Athletes' mental health, performance, and development. *International Journal of Sport and Exercise Psychology 16*(6), 622–639. https://doi.org/10.1080/1612197X.2017.1295557.

Vieira, L. F., Rodacki, A. L. F., Caruzzo, N. M., Moreira, C. R., Contreira, A. R., Lima, Fortes, L. S., Vissoci, J. R. N., & Stefanello, J. M. (2019). Sport and exercise psychology studies in Brazil: Performance or health? *Frontiers in Psychology 10*, 1–10. http://doi.org/10.3389/fpsyg.2019.02154.

Welsh, E. (2002). Dealing with data: Using NVivo in the qualitative data analysis process. *Forum Qualitative Sozialforschung 3*(2). https://doi.org/10.17169/fqs-3.2.865.

Wood, S., Harrison, L. K., & Kucharska, J. (2017). Male professional footballers' experiences of mental health difficulties and help-seeking. *The Physician and Sports Medicine 45*(2), 120–128. http://dx.doi.org/10.1080/00913847.2017.1283209.

5

ESTABLISHING A MENTAL HEALTH CLINIC FOR ELITE SPORTS

The Swedish model

Göran Kenttä and Karin Hyland

Context – and background

In brief, elite sport in Sweden is supported by three overarching umbrella organizations, the Swedish Paralympic committee, the Swedish Olympics committee and the Swedish Sport Confederations elite sport department. Each organization has a small number of employed sport psychologists (SP), which are practitioners trained in both traditional performance enhancement and psychotherapy with a clinical education to provide sport psychology services to elite athletes. Minor mental health problems that go beyond performance enhancement issues are treated by these employees. In cases of more serious clinical disorders, athletes belonging to a national team (or having recently retired) and being over 18 years of age can access one of the two Clinics for Mental Health and Elite Sports in Stockholm or Malmö. The same conditions apply to elite coaches.

Elite sport in Sweden largely share the global culture of high performance sport (Olusoga & Kenttä, 2017). The stigma and denial of mental illness in athletes have been a shared attitude in the domain of elite sports (Schwenk, 2000), including Sweden. Attributes such as mental strength, mental toughness, grit, and resilience are highly desirable characteristics in elite sports in contrast to mental illness and help-seeking that is associated to vulnerability and mental weakness (Gulliver, Griffiths, & Christensen, 2012). As a consequence, when suffering, instead of showing any sign of weakness and vulnerability we rather tend to "put on a smile on our face and continue to be successful – but when mission is completed we go home and feel like shit" (words from one client).

Gulliver and colleagues (2012) described reasons behind why elite athletes don't seek help for mental health problems; it is stigma around mental health problems, there is a lack of knowledge and understanding about mental health, help-seeking is perceived as a sign of weakness and mental health is not linked to performance. This high threshold for help-seeking is troublesome and put athletes at the risk of developing more severe conditions.

Interestingly, when successful world class athletes from sports that typically represent a masculine and macho stereotype open up and share personal stories of vulnerability it seems to reduce the threshold for help-seeking. Tyson Fury, a heavyweight boxing champion, has been

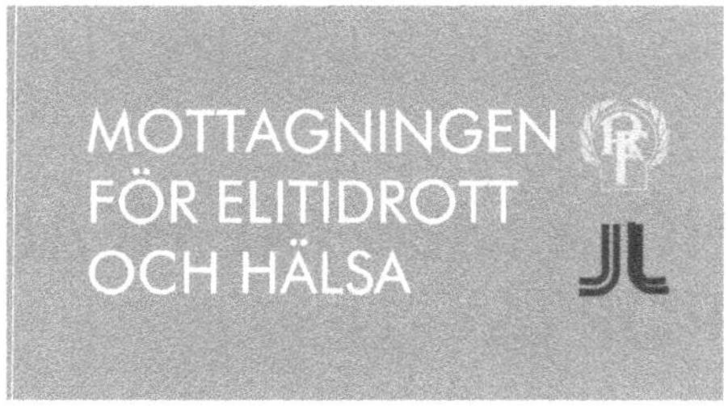

FIGURE 5.1 Physical sign RGI

open with his severe depression and today he says: "Seek help! That is the message that I'd love to spread a million times." Sir John James Patrick Kirwan played for New Zealand from 1984 until 1994. He played a major role in the All Blacks' 23 test unbeaten run from 1987 to 1990, including winning the 1987 World Cup. Kirwan has openly spoken of his battle with depression, and is actively involved in mental health and depression awareness campaigns in New Zealand. He has written about his depression in the books *All Blacks Don't Cry* and *Stand by Me*. Kirwan showcase how athletes can maintain a high level of success in spite of a coexistent primary psychiatric disorder as suggested by Reardon and Factor (2010). These examples may serve as ambassadors and their message can potentially make it easier for athletes that suffer to actually seek psychiatric care.

Case: "Riddargatan 1 – The Mental Health Clinic for Elite Sports"

The mental health clinic will be described by the overall purpose, how it operates, that includes staff, eligible criteria´s, intake, assessment, who is the patient, treatment, and the aim to serve as a knowledge hub. In February 2015 "Riddargatan 1 – The Mental Health Clinic for Elite Sports" opened. This is an outpatient clinic located in Stockholm and part of the Stockholm Center for Dependency Disorders. Since the start, the overall purpose has been to provide high-quality health care specifically to elite level athletes and coaches. In order to do this, the aim has been to be generously available to identify needs, assess, treat, and better understand mental disorders and related problems in elite sports.

Purpose and challenges at the start

Before the start it was important to agree upon the following statements that did answer the key question: Why do we need a specialist clinic for mental health disorders that target elite sports?

- ✓ Give attention to previously unmet clinical treatment needs (in large contrast to available sports medicine support)
- ✓ Lower the threshold for help-seeking by reducing stigma regarding mental health problems and by normalizing mental health problems
- ✓ Prevent long term ill-being by early treatment
- ✓ Provide high quality care (assessment and treatment) in a multidisciplinary team
- ✓ Gather knowledge about the prevalence of specific disorders
- ✓ Become a knowledge-hub

✓ Acknowledge that also successful athletes and coaches in high performance sports mirror the general population in prevalence of mental health disorders

Among the statements above, the first one, was by far the most important reason to go from thought to action. It was important to address what was identified as unmet treatment demands among elite level athletes and coaches suffering from mental health problems. Moreover, there is currently no indication that mental health problems will decline in society or elite sports.

This clinic, basically started from scratch, being the first of its kind in Sweden, and most likely also being the first of its kind globally, where publicly financed healthcare and a National Sports Confederation collaborate. On one hand it was truly a start from scratch; on the other hand, this specialist clinic was embedded in one of the largest dependency clinics in Europe with about 700 employees and about 20,000 patients receiving treatment with about 350,000 sessions every year. Internet based psychotherapy has recently increased. This was a resource of expertise and experience. The clinic is located in the city center of Stockholm, close to public transportations and is housed in a multi-business building making the visit more discrete for personal integrity. These values, specifically lowering the threshold for help-seeking and providing professional and discrete care at an early stage, did resonate with those of the National Sport Confederation.

Since the start we have been treating elite athletes (over the age of 18 years) and their coaches from various Swedish national teams with mental health problems like stress and exhaustion syndrome/burnout, social anxiety, OCD, PTSD, GAD, panic disorder, eating disorders, affective disorders, self-harm, and suicidal behavior, dependence disorders, ADHD, autism spectrum disorders, and performance issues.

There were a lot of doubts, some harsh criticism and skepticism at the start. People questioned if any high level athlete or coach actually need and would seek psychiatric care. It was basically impossible to predict any number of care-seekers or the severity of disorders (i.e., complexity and length of treatment) before the start. Altogether, it was necessary for the stakeholders to take a stance and to be humble and accept all the uncertainty at the start. Consequently, it was decided that the first year started as a pilot that should be carefully evaluated. After the first year the number of care-seekers was pretty small, however, it was noticeable that their psychiatric problems were complex and the feedback regarding treatment was positive. As a result, it was decided by the stakeholders that the clinic did serve a purpose and it became permanent and, more importantly, it was allowed to grow organically. Now after five years, the clinic can be considered established and fulfill an important need. Having key persons in leading positions from both organizations that did believe in this pioneering project at the start was crucial.

Staff

As previously noted, the clinic has had the advantage of being able to grow organically due to the need for psychiatric care. Moreover, this was also related to hiring staff that would create a dream team at the start. At the beginning a senior consultant in psychiatry, with broad experience from psychiatric care, worked part-time together with one licensed psychologist and (sport psychology) CBT-therapists specifically trained to work with both clinical and performance issues in elite sports and with extensive experience in performance issues.

The whole idea is to strive both for mental well-being and retained performance. After some organic growth, today there are six staff members; two experienced senior consultants in psychiatry, two licensed psychologists, and two (sport psychology) CBT-therapists working together as a multidisciplinary team at the clinic. Importantly, the psychiatrist is the only profession that is fully eligible to prescribe and provide pharmacological treatment in addition to issue certificates needed for sick-leave. Moreover, certificates to The World Anti-Doping Agency (WADA) is needed when medicine is on the prohibited list. Noteworthy, the psychologists are all trained in Cognitive Behavioral Therapy (CBT) and the last wave of CBT. Acceptance- and mindfulness based therapies is a shared knowledge and approach among all staff members.

Eligible criteria's

Interestingly, in hindsight, setting the eligible criteria before the start was one of the first challenges to collaborate between the world of sports and psychiatry. The latter with strict and less flexible systems including law and justice that is a basic condition for any public health care system. In comparison, the world of elite sports focus on performance and seem to have several blurred boundaries in regard of psychological support.

More specifically, to have access to any clinic that operates within adult psychiatry, three explicit eligible criteria need to be fulfilled. At first, the athlete (i.e., the patient) needs to be above 18 years of age. Under 18 years of age, child and adolescent psychiatry is the available choice according to the Swedish healthcare system. Secondly, the patient (i.e., the athlete) personally need to seek help. Thirdly, the patient (i.e., the athlete) need to fulfill at least one psychiatric diagnosis in order to be eligible to receive treatment. Importantly, the care system allows a Swedish citizen to seek care anywhere in the country no matter residential address.

At first, the sports criteria's may look just as clear, being a current elite level athlete, or a recently retired athlete. However, simply setting a clear criterion for an elite athlete is challenging (Swann, Moran, & Piggott, 2015), and even more so for a coach. Finally, we did agree upon setting the criteria to have been at a national team at least once during the last two years. Since this was a collaboration between public health care and NGB of sports, only sports that were organized and part of the Swedish Sport Confederation were included. This means that sports such as cross-fit, body-building, and e-sport were excluded. The time period for recently retired was set to 12 months. Exclusion criteria were having an on-going treatment contact in psychiatry elsewhere, just wanting a second opinion or being a citizen outside of Sweden.

Intake

In order to attend to the clinic, the athletes and coaches first log on to a website and fill in an application form and shortly describe their current problems. This is a common procedure used by the public health care system. They also provide a phone number for communication. If the athlete or coach has had an engagement in a Swedish national team during the last two years and have no current psychiatric treatment a decision is made to contact the athlete to schedule an appointment. To provide the urgent service that elite sports require, it has been important to handle applications as fast as possible. In practice, most applicants have been scheduled to the first appointment within a week from their application.

Assessment

The first appointment is always a face-to-face meeting. The patient meets a psychiatrist who makes an assessment that also includes the Mini International Neuropsychiatric Interview (MINI; Sheedan et al., 1998), plus a clinical assessment (Clinical Global Impression Scale; Busner & Targum, 2007). The MINI is a brief structured diagnostic interview that assesses the 17 most common disorders in mental health. Web based questionnaires for initial self-assessment are completed by all care seekers, ideally before the first appointment. Symptoms of anxiety and depression are assessed with Hospital Anxiety and Depression Scale (HADS; Zigmond & Snaith, 1983) and Patient Health Questionnaire (PHQ-9; Spitzer, Kroenke, & Williams, 1999). Severity of hazardous drinking is assessed with Alcohol Use Disorders Identification Test for Consumption (AUDIT-C; Gordon et al., 2001). The adult ADHD Self-Report Scale screener (ASRS screener) is used to screen for adult attention-deficit/hyperactivity disorder (Kessler et al., 2005). The EQ5D-5L questionnaire measure health related quality of life (Herdman, et al., 2011) and the 12-item World Health Organization Disability Assessment Schedule (WHODAS 2.0) asks about difficulties due to health conditions (Rehm et al., 1999). The athletes also fill in self-assessments regarding performance and a standardized scale assessing psychological flexibility (AAQ; Bond et al., 2011), that typically is a goal in treatment. All self-assessment questionnaires are also filled in after treatment completion and symptom specific questionnaires are used during treatment when clinically appropriate. Diagnose specific self-reports might be used as complement when needed. The assessment includes biomarkers in blood when considered relevant and sometimes a somatic examination by a general practitioner is needed. The different parts of the assessment results most often in one or more diagnoses. In fact, a very limited number of help-seekers have not fulfilled a clinical diagnose. Moreover, a psychologist or a sport psychologist also assesses the new patient with a focus on a functional behavioral analysis in order to better understand the behavioral aspect related to the mental health problem. The next step is a multidisciplinary team discussion about the diagnoses and an appropriate treatment plan. Performance issues are always an integral part during the process of assessment and treatment. Each case is discussed with special attention to the relationship between treatment, sport specific training, and competition. The team provides feedback to the patient the same day or shortly after the two appointments. The feedback includes the current diagnoses and the patients are offered treatment when needed. The treatment plan is worked out and updated regularly during the treatment. It is common to involve coaches, parents, or other important persons in the treatment as long as the patient agrees to this. No information can be shared to others, unless the patient gives his or her consent, due to health care confidentiality.

Who is the patient?

About 330 individuals have received support during the first five years. Most of the athletes are young, between 18 and 30 years, and the coaches are older. A majority reside in the region of Stockholm, but about 40% comes from cities outside of Stockholm representing most parts of Sweden. There a balance between male and female athletes. Many athletes seek help after pro-long periods or repeated bouts of injury. For the majority this is the first contact with specialized psychiatrisy, while others have previous experience. Very few have experience from pharmacological treatment. It is quite common to have worked with a sport psychologist regarding performance issues and sometimes the sport psychologist refers the patient to the clinic. This is mostly the case for athletes, but sometimes also the case for coaches. However, there are a greater variety behind athletes' initiative to contact the clinic, for example through physiotherapists, nutritionists, club coaches, National Team coaches, parents, and the patients themselves. In addition, there is also a greater variety of diagnoses among athletes as compared to coaches. Coaches predominately present depression, exhaustion, and substance use disorders as their prime diagnosis, with limited cases of eating disorders, performance anxiety, panic syndrome, and PTSD that are more frequently presented by athletes. Finally, signposting a way to find mental health support is important. Two recent initiatives have addressed this challenge. A new health care system was launched as a digital application in May 2019 by the Swedish Sport Confederation. However, primarily to guide care-seekers to sports medicine support, but there is also a possibility to request psychiatric care. By the end of 2019 it was accessible by about 5000 national team level athletes in Sweden. Another initiative was to build and launch a web-site including the mental health literacy and clear links to the two mental health clinics. It is too early to evaluate the impact of these two initiatives.

Treatment

Most patients who have passed the threshold and actually do seek help are typically committed and engaged in treatment. Treatment always have a strong foundation in evidence based CBT. It is important to note that about 25–30 percent of the patients are given pharmacological treatment in addition to CBT. Anti-depressants are the most common drugs used. Other examples are pharmacological treatment for sleeping disorders and ADHD. The most common disorders treated are different anxiety disorders including performance anxiety, depression, stress, and exhaustion syndrome/burnout and various types of eating disorders. Most often there are more than one diagnoses to consider. It is not uncommon that more diagnoses become obvious later, e.g., when the therapeutic alliance grow stronger and the patient become more comfortable to share their suffering or when an extended assessment is made when ADHD is likely to be the underlying explanation to the current symptoms.

The CBT given follows the appropriate protocols for the different diagnoses such as the intolerance of uncertainty model by Robichaud and Dugas (2006) for General Anxiety Disorder, the CBT-E according to Fairburn (2008) for eating disorders and behavioral activation model for depression by Martell and colleagues (2013). Moreover, Acceptance and Commitment Therapy (ACT), mindfulness and self-compassion are common ingredients in the psychological treatment. The number of sessions with CBT differs a lot, and so does time in treatment. Median number of sessions are about 12 sessions, if the 10% of patients that have been in treatment more than 30 sessions are excluded. A session is typically about 45 minutes. Noteworthy, there is not a strictly fixed number of sessions. The length and frequency of treatment is decided in collaboration with the client and the treatment team with respect to the identified need often including the competitive schedule. During the treatment the team and the patient have common team conferences together to evaluate the treatment plan. When relevant, important others also cooperate in these conferences and evaluations. When the goals according to the treatment plan are achieved we prepare for the end of the contact. The same self-assessment questionnaires that were used initially are filled in and the treatment given is evaluated by the patient and the team together. Here we learn a lot from the patients´ perceptions of what was helpful in the treatment.

A knowledge hub with research and practice

Staff members have presented at several international conferences, national meetings covering specific sport federation, sport psychology, and sports medicine meetings. A doctoral student is also attached to the clinic. The clinic has also been open and welcoming Nordic and other international collaborations.

Reflections – lessons learned

At first it can be concluded that there is still a need to better support mental health issues and thereby enhance sustainability in elite sports. Following this, it can also be concluded that psychiatric issues in relationship to performance represent a complex and dynamic relationship.

Why did it take so long?

From one perspective we think that stakeholders, organizations, academic scholars, and practitioners in Sweden and elsewhere need to question themselves, why did it take so long to acknowledge and direct attention to mental health and psychiatry in the context of elite sports? Why did it take until 2015 to open up a specialized clinic in psychiatry for elite sports and mental health? Why did it take until 2018 to publish the first comprehensive position statement on elite sports and mental health? Interestingly, this was followed by another 5–6 position statements within two years. Sadly, but also importantly, there are examples of tragic stories that alert the attention and need for mental health initiatives. In Sweden, Mikael Ljungberg a beloved and cherished high profile wrestler, an Olympic gold medalist and two times winner of the world championships, committed suicide in November 2004 when the readiness to fully engage in mental health support did not exist.

Sustainability

Sustainability in any system, ultimately depends on demands and supply. No demands, effort would be a waste. However, all signs in research and practice speak for a lasting demand of mental health support and psychiatric service that also target elite sport. It is therefore argued that maintaining resources is the key challenge. In this case, our described specialist psychiatric clinic fully depends on continued support from key stakeholders that authorize support to maintain professional service to athletes and coaches. In order to maintain professional service at a specialist clinic staff is essential. More specifically, as noted by Lebrun and Collins (2017), when working with elite athletes and high performance coaches and their mental health there is need for practitioners with a dual competence. First and foremost, clinical expertise is needed, but also a contextual knowledge and understanding of high performance sport that is important when dealing with diagnostic and therapeutic challenges relative to mental health and performance issues. Managing the need for these dual competences and skills will be further addressed from different perspectives.

Performance vs. clinical treatment

It was previously concluded that psychiatric issues in relationship to performance represents a complex and dynamic relationship. Another challenge integrated into this complexity is a conflicting interest between traditional psychiatry that primarily focuses on clinical treatment and the support system developed for elite sport that primarily focus on performance. On one hand, it can be argued that success in treatment in our case should include two outcome measures, (1) increased or maintained functioning in sports (i.e., performance related outcomes) and (2) reduction in clinical symptoms (i.e., diagnostic related outcomes). On the other hand, it can be argued that the overriding psychiatric treatment goal always should prioritize reduced suffering. On a more complex note, there have been individual cases that after treatment reach a high-degree of well-being but also decide to drop-out of sports. Should this be regarded as a failure in treatment? A common personality characteristic among a number of clients at the clinic can be described as clinical perfectionism, expressed by self-worth that is dependent on success and achievement and when underperforming having a highly self-critical inner voice that pushes to work harder. This is a strong, but also a "dark" driving force behind excessive training and an athletic success. It is typically a fear to let go of this driving force, but it can also lead to a sense of freedom and realization that it is time to also leave elite sports. Acceptance and commitment approaches specifically giving attention to values have been important in several challenging cases. This approach emphasizes the athlete to focus on their current situation and take appropriate action toward achieving their goals and values, even in the presence of challenging or unwanted psychological events (e.g., thoughts, feelings, physiological sensations, images, and memories).

On a final note, finding a balanced way to give appropriate attention to both mental health and performance is key, but also challenging. This balanced approach, means that at times it can be ok to give priority to performance if there is major competition, and at time give priority to mental health because suffering limits functioning in all areas of life including sport.

Sport specific or generic models of care

Psychiatry and clinical psychology typical apply evidence based generic treatment models. However, Rice and colleagues (2016) argued that sport specific treatment models should be developed. Overall the experience is that athletes and coaches with diagnosis such as depression, dependency disorders, OCD, GAD, panic syndromes, and PTSD adapt well to standardized treatment protocols that exist in psychiatric care. However, it should be noted that adapting the treatment to the context of elite sports is largely beneficial. For example, behavioral activation with a depressed athlete can be to adhere to the rehab program when injured that is prescribed by a physio according to a weekly set schedule, or finding positive reinforcement in an individual training session when dropping performance demands.

In contrast to the more generic models of care, it is suggested that exhaustion syndrome/burnout, anxiety related to performance anxiety and eating disorders are more sensitive to a sport specific context and would benefit from more sport specific models of care. For example is important to examine the cause behind an athlete that present severe exhaustion that can be related to excessive training, life stressors, and or inadequate recovery. Being able to address and discuss recovery related to the sport specific context and regular demands in training is important. Eating disorders may by the most sensitive issue for several reasons. At times, it enhances performance, it is contagious between athletes, and it is associated with high risk of health. Ultimately, the most difficult challenge is related to making a decision to stop an athlete from training and competing, and then consequently later in treatment also decide when it is time to "return to play." With an open collaboration with the athletes and their coaches a gradual return to training can be made in a way that is advantageous.

Moreover, in many aesthetic sports (such as gymnastsics, figure skating, synchronized swimming), weightbearing sports (such as middle-distance running, triathlon, road cycling, and cross-country skiing) and weight class sports (boxing, wrestling and rowing) there is more and more attention toward weight regulation with an aim to strive toward a magic optimal body weight. Perhaps more attention needs to focus on responsible weight regulation in a similar manner as responsible drinking in treatment of alcohol, responsible gambling in treatment of gambling disorders and responsible return after concussion. On a final note, we state that contextual knowledge is essential and can never be underestimated when working with elite athletes and high performance coaches.

Multidisciplinary treatment and collaborative learning

It first needs to be stated firmly. At the start, no multidisciplinary model included sport psychology, clinical psychology, and psychiatry within the public health care system. Thus, it was basically a blank start. Moreover, psychiatry and clinical psychology is strictly confidential and compared to sports medicine less integrated into both theory and practice of elite sports (i.e., not at all). Sport psychiatry is rare in high performance sports despite a profession that is specialized in assessment and treatment of mental disorders. For a specific example, the Olympic and Paralympic village include a comprehensively equipped clinic that host a range of practitioners in sports medicine, but extremely limited in psychiatry. In contrast to sport psychology support that often is totally integrated in the context and almost without boundaries, psychiatry is strictly regulated by professional secrecy.

Finding and organizing opportunities to learn organically within the multidisciplinary team, and identifying knowledge gaps and learning needs in a prestige-less manner, have been fundamentally important. Initiatives to do this are bi-weekly multidisciplinary meetings and monthly sessions with and external supervisor with a focus on the most challenging cases. In addition, several experts have been invited to lunch seminars to cover topics such as eating disorder, sports medicine, and concussion. The team also regularly attend external workshops together on topics such as acceptance and commitment therapy, self-compassion, and health anxiety. Finally, attending and finding learning opportunities with an emphasis on more strict performance psychology has been important. Altogether, these efforts support a greater understanding, knowledge, and respect between the professions that are ultimately important to strengthen professional boundaries as well as a collaborative multidisciplinary team.

Future directions

It is suggested that the last three topics discussed would benefit from future research. More specifically, give attention to; (I) the complex relationship between clinical treatment and performance issues; (II) sport specific models of care, and (III) the collaborative learning process in a multidisciplinary treatment team. The last topic should be addressed by potential barriers and supportive factors when comparing one physical location, a virtual team, and possibly a combination of the two.

References

Åkesdotter, C., Kenttä, G., Eloranta, S., & Franck, J. (2020). The prevalence of Mental Health Problems in elite athletes. *Journal of Science and Medicine in Sport 23*, 329–335.

Bond, F.W., Hayes, S. C., Bear, R. A., et al. (2011). Preliminary psychometric properties of the Acceptance and Action Questionnaire – II: A revised measure of psychological inflexibility and experiential avoidance, *Behavior Therapy 42*, 676–688.

Busner, J., & Targum, S. D. (2007). Clinical Global Impression Scale: Applying a research tool in clinical practice, *Psychiatry* 7, 28–37.

Fairburn, C. G. (2008). *Cognitive Behavior Therapy and Eating Disorders*. Guilford Press. London.

Gordon, A. J., Maisto, S. A., McNeil, M., Kraemer, K. L., Conigliaro, R. L., Kelley, M. E., & Conigliaro, J. (2001). Three questions can detect hazardous drinkers. *The Journal of Family Practice 4*, 313–320.

Gulliver, A., Griffiths, K. M., & Christensen, H. (2012). Barriers and facilitators to mental health help-seeking for young elite athletes: A qualitative study. *BMC Psychiatry 12*, 157–171.

Henriksen, K., Schinke, R., Moesch, K., McCann, S., Parham, W. D., Larsen, C. H., & Terry, P. (2019). Consensus statement on improving the mental health of high performance athletes. *International Journal of Sport and Exercise Psychology*.

Herdman, M., Gudex, C., Lloyd, A., et al. (2011). Development and preliminary testing of the new five-level version of EQ-5D (EQ-5D-5L). *Quality of Life Research 20*, 1727–1736.

Kessler, R. C., Adler, L., Ames, M., et al. (2005). The World Health Organization Adult ADHD Self-Report Scale (ASRS): A short screening scale for use in the general population. *Psychological Medicine 35*, 245–256.

Kirwan, John (2010). *All Blacks don't cry: A story of hope*. Penguin. North Shore, N.Z.

Lebrun, F., & Collins, D. (2017). Is elite sport (really) bad for you? Can we answer the question? *Frontiers in Psychology 8*, 324.

Martell, C. R., Dimidjian, S., & Herman-Dunn, R. (2013). *Behavioral activations model for depression: A clinicians' guide*. The Guilford Press. New York, NY.

Moesch, K., Kenttä, G., Kleinert, J., Quignon-Fleuret, C., Cecil, S., & Bertollo, M. (2018). FEPSAC position statement: Mental health disorders in elite athletes and models of service provision. *Psychology of Sport and Exercise 38*, 61–71.

Olusoga, P., & Kenttä, G. (2017). Desperate to quit: A narrative analysis of burnout and recovery in high performance sports coaching. *The Sport Psychologist 3*, 237–248.

Reardon, C. L., & Factor, R. M. (2010). Sport psychiatry. A systematic review of diagnoses and medical treatment of mental illness in athletes. *Sports Medicine, 40*, 961–980.

Reardon, C. L., Hainline, B., Aron, C. M., Baron, D., Baum, A. L., Bindra, A., … Engebretsen, L. (2019). Mental health in elite athletes: International Olympic Committee consensus statement (2019). *British Journal of Sports Medicine 53*, 667–699.

Rehm, J., Ustun, T. B., Saxena, S., et al. (1999). On the development and psychometric testing of the WHO screening instrument to assess disablement in the general population. *International Journal of Methods in Psychiatric Research 8*, 110–122.

Rice, S. M., Purcell, R., De Silva, S., Mawren, D., McGorry, P., & Parker, A. G. (2016). The mental health of elite athletes: A narrative systematic review. *Sports Medicine 49*, 1333–1353.

Robichaud, M., & Dugas, M. J. (2006). A cognitive-behavioral treatment targeting intolerance of uncertainty. In G. C. L. Davey & A. Wells (Eds.). *Worry and its psychological disorders: Theory, assessment and treatment* (pp. 289–304). John Wiley & Sons Ltd. Chichester, UK.

Schinke, R. J., Stambulova, N. B., Si, G., & Moore, Z. (2018). International society of sport psychology position stand: Athletes' mental health, performance, and development. *International Journal of Sport and Exercise Psychology 6*, 622–639.

Schwenk, T. L. (2000), The stigmatisation and denial of mental illness in athletes. *British Journal of Sports Medicine 34*, 4–5.

Sheehan, D.V., Lecrubier, Y., Harnett-Sheehan, K., et al. (1998). The Mini International Neuropsychiatric Interview (M.I.N.I.): The Development and Validation of a Structured Diagnostic Psychiatric Interview. *Journal of Clinical Psychiatry 59(suppl.20)*, 22–33.

Spitzer, R. L., Kroenke, K., & Williams, J. B. W. (1999). Validation and utility of a self-report version of PRIME-MD: The PHQ Primary Care Study. *Journal of the American Medical Association 282*, 1737–1744.

Steel, Z., Marnane, C., Iranpour, C., et al. (2014). The global prevalence of common mental disorders: A systematic review and meta-analysis 1980–2013. *International Journal of Epidemiology 2*, 476–493.

Swann, C. H., Moran, A., & Piggott, D. (2015). Defining elite athletes: Issues in the study of expert performance in sport psychology. *Psychology of Sport and Exercise 16*, 3–14.

Van Slingerland, K., Durand-Bush, N., Bradley, L., Goldfield, G., Archambault, R., Smith, D., Edwards, C., Delenardo, S., Taylor, S., Werthner, P., & Kenttä, G. (2019). Canadian Centre for Mental Health and Sport (CCMHS) position statement: Principles of mental health in competitive and high-performance sport. *Clinical Journal of Sport Medicine 29*, 173–180.

Zigmond, A. S., & Snaith, R. P. (1983). The hospital anxiety and depression scale. *Acta Psychiatrica Scandinavica 67*, 361–370.

6

CREATING A NATIONAL SYSTEM TO SUPPORT MENTAL HEALTH AND ENHANCE WELL-BEING ACROSS HIGH PERFORMANCE SPORT

Lisa Olive, Simon Rice, Matt Butterworth, Mary Spillane, Matti Clements, and Rosemary Purcell

Who we are

This case study is authored by practicing mental health clinician-researchers in clinical psychology, social work, as well as leaders in the sports and youth mental health sectors. In presenting this case, we draw on our expertise, as well as international experience in global mental health initiatives, including a mental health partnership with the World Economic Forum (Orygen, 2019), and as co-authors of the International Olympic Committee's Expert Consensus Statement on Elite Athlete Mental Health (Reardon et al., 2019).

As authors situated across two nation-wide Australian organizations – the Australian Institute of Sport (AIS), and Orygen's Elite Sport and Mental Health Program (co-affiliated with the Centre for Youth Mental Health, The University of Melbourne) – our perspectives canvass both the elite sport sector and the provision of early intervention through to specialist mental health care and service models. The AIS is Australia's peak high performance sport agency that supports National Sporting Organizations (NSOs) and their athletes to achieve their highest potential. Orygen is Australia's leading organization in youth mental health and early intervention, combining both research and clinical services to young people, to enhance knowledge translation on mental ill-health in young people (www.orygen.org.au). In reflecting on the rationale for, and implementation of, the AIS's Mental Health Referral Network, this chapter offers a roadmap and critique of the initiative from the team of clinicians responsible for its initial establishment. In doing so, this chapter aims to provide reflections on key lessons learned to provide guidance for international bodies seeking to embark on similar comprehensive athlete mental health and well-being support systems.

Mental health in elite sports: Establishing the need for a system response

Emerging evidence in elite athlete mental health is shaping a narrative that indicates that poor mental health is common among athletes, at a level at, or even exceeding, the general population (Markser, 2011; S. M. Rice et al., 2016). However, a number of important gaps still exist in our knowledge, which limits the ability to draw firm conclusions regarding the prevalence and nature of mental health conditions in currently competing elite athletes and how best to develop a response to address athlete needs. To address this knowledge gap, AIS Athlete Wellbeing and Engagement, in collaboration with Orygen's Elite Sport and Mental Health program, developed and conducted in 2018 the AIS Mental Health Audit. This was an anonymous online survey, designed to better understand the mental health and well-being needs of National Sporting Organization (NSO) categorized athletes in Australia.

The AIS Mental Health Audit

What was measured?

Survey assessments included measures of *mental health symptoms* (e.g., anxiety, depression, social dysfunction, and somatic symptoms) and *probable caseness*, the latter defined as symptoms that adversely affect quality of life and which are of a level frequently found among individuals seeking help from health professionals (Goldberg et al., 1997). Further assessments included measures of *psychological distress*, *maladaptive response to psychological distress*, *gambling behavior*, *risky alcohol consumption*, *self-esteem*, *body weight and shape dissatisfaction*, *satisfaction with life*, *adverse life events*, *social support*, *help seeking*, *coping style*, and finally, a measure to control for *socially desirable responding*. (For a more detailed description of the assessments involved in the survey, see Purcell, Rice, Butterworth, & Clements, 2020.)

Based on the knowledge that a wide array of risk factors are associated with increased vulnerability to mental health symptoms, including (but not limited to) genetic, biological, and environmental factors (Arango et al., 2018), the survey also assessed a number of potential correlates. These were broadly categorized as demographic characteristics (e.g., age, gender, sexuality, education), individual-vulnerability factors (e.g., perceived adequacy of social support, coping style, adverse life events, history of treatment for a psychological or mental health problem), and sports-related factors (e.g., injury status, concussion, individual vs. team sport, recent major competition, length of elite sporting career).

What was found?

A total of 1566 athletes (16.0% athletes from para-sports) aged 17 years and older (mean age 24.5 years) were registered with the AIS at the time of the survey and eligible to participate (52.5% male; 47.5% female). Of these, 810 consented to participate (51.7% response rate) and valid data was available from 749 athletes. The participating athletes were representative of the eligible population in relation to their mean age (24.6 years) and para-status (14.7%), although a higher proportion of female athletes completed the survey (54.1%).

The results indicated that the rates of psychological distress and probable 'caseness' in the month prior to the survey were higher among athletes than community norms, with almost one in five athletes reporting 'high to very high' psychological distress and one in three reporting mental health symptoms at a level that would usually warrant treatment by a health professional (i.e., caseness). Despite elevated rates of psychological distress and caseness, athletes conversely reported better body satisfaction, life satisfaction, and self-esteem than community norms, and lower rates of risky alcohol consumption and lower problem gambling. Athletes reporting higher levels of psychological distress and probable caseness also reported a greater number of recent adverse events, but these factors were not correlated with injury status.

The most robust correlates of mental health outcomes in this cohort were demographic and individual-vulnerability factors, particularly recent treatment for a mental health or psychological problem, the adequacy of social support and coping styles. It is important to note that each of these factors are dynamic and modifiable, not only at the individual level (e.g., by developing more adaptive coping skills) but also at organizational levels. For example, lifting policies that limit or ban partners/family from attending major competitions and creating sporting environments in which athletes feel safe to disclose and seek treatment for their mental health symptoms represent two modifications to address these factors.

The correlates of alcohol consumption differed, being positively associated with team sports, as well as working in paid fulltime employment (in addition to their elite sporting career) and negatively associated with female gender, being a para-athlete and completion of higher levels of education. The audit findings also suggest that the odds of caseness were associated with having been treated for a concussion and/or a psychological problem, and also experiencing multiple concussions. This is an area of research that warrants further investigation given that prior research has indicated an association between concussion exposure and depressive symptoms in elite athletes (Rice et al., 2018).

The AIS Mental Health Audit is the first study to examine the rates of mental health symptoms in a large, national representative sample of currently contracted elite athletes, inclusive of gender and para-athlete status, and to compare observed rates to population norms or representative community samples. The findings highlight the critical need for elite sports organizations, and the professionals who work with them, to support athletes, to recognize that a significant proportion of athletes are likely to experience mental health symptoms and may require clinical care to manage their symptoms and restore optimal mental health and functioning. With one in five athletes in this sample reporting having previously sought treatment for a mental health or psychological problem, the need for models of mental health care that are able to identify and respond to athlete mental health needs, while also considering the unique aspects that an elite sporting context brings with it is apparent. In the next section, we outline the AIS's response to these findings and the innovations made to mental health care in the Australian elite sporting context.

The context: The Australian Institute of Sport

The AIS is Australia's peak high performance sport agency that seeks to lead and enable a united, collaborative high performance system that supports athletes to achieve podium success. The AIS is the high performance branch of the Australian Sports Commission, an Australian Government affiliation that supports, develops and invests in sport at all levels, from community participation to elite athletes. The AIS provides leadership, coordination, and support for high performance sport. It administers funding for; high-performance and national programs, research and innovation, and its two campuses on behalf of the Australian Government.

Historical context of the AIS

The AIS was built in 1981 in response to the 1976 Montreal Olympic campaign where Australia did not win a single gold medal. The AIS was conceived to be an innovative problem-solver for Australian sport, bringing together a critical mass of sports scientists, coaches, administrators, and athletes in a centralized daily training environment. At its conception, the AIS was unique in Australia, drawing on ideas from established sports institutes in Europe, but has since become a common model adopted around the world.

Since its inception, the AIS has undergone significant change and reform. Once a lone centralized institute located in Canberra, Australia, with the majority of sports (and their athletes) located locally or on-site at the AIS, during the mid-to-late 80s, each Australian state established independent sports institutes and academies (now known as the National Institute Network [NIN]) in response to demands for a *decentralized* system. Recent changes have resulted in a decentralized system of the AIS itself, working alongside the NIN, where a greater emphasis has been placed on the NSOs to govern the use of resources and funding from Sport Australia. One of the challenges of moving from a centralized model, where sports science and sports medicine (SSSM; e.g., exercise physiology, dietetics and nutrition, sports psychology and mental health, biomechanics) were all centrally located and their services readily delivered in the daily training environment, has been the need to develop approaches to athlete management that could now cater to athletes spread across the country and internationally. In addition to these changes, when it came to psychological service delivery at the AIS, historically, the emphasis was placed on performance, which was reflected in a workforce that mainly comprised sports psychologists. It was not until 2005 that the first clinical psychologist was instated to oversee the well-being of residential and AIS affiliated athletes. Since this time, the AIS has identified the need for, and invested heavily in, the provision of mental health services and supports for its affiliated athletes.

AIS Athlete Wellbeing and Engagement

In response to the decentralization of the AIS, the newly formed AIS Athlete Wellbeing and Engagement team was established in 2018. This team is tasked with leading and supporting each NSO to create cultures where they can support athletes to find the right balance between well-being, engagement in activities outside of training and competition, and the requirements of elite sport. The Athlete Wellbeing and Engagement program focuses on five key domains: career and education, community engagement, conduct and professionalism (including ethical decision making around athlete safety and well-being), personal development, and mental health (see Figure 6.1). These five focus domains were identified by a specialist team of AIS staff, who are also responsible for leading and implementing the service provision that addresses each specific area. This has been achieved with the support of the NSOs and the NIN, where a network of Athlete Wellbeing and Engagement Managers, directly employed by, and embedded in their NSO or NIN, has been established. The NSO/NIN based Athlete Wellbeing and Engagement Managers have a core responsibility to their NSO or NIN to implement the Athlete Wellbeing and Engagement strategy that their organization has developed in partnership with the AIS. In doing so, the Athlete Wellbeing and Engagement program seeks to enable holistic athlete development, promoting the athletic and non-athletic skills that athletes need to live a productive life.

Key to supporting and maintaining positive athlete mental health is the timely provision and access to evidence-based intervention, as appropriate. In response to this aim, the AIS Athlete Wellbeing and Engagement established a dedicated Mental Health Team to prioritize and strengthen athlete mental health through an athlete-centric support model. At the centerpiece of this unit has been the development of the Mental Health Referral Network.

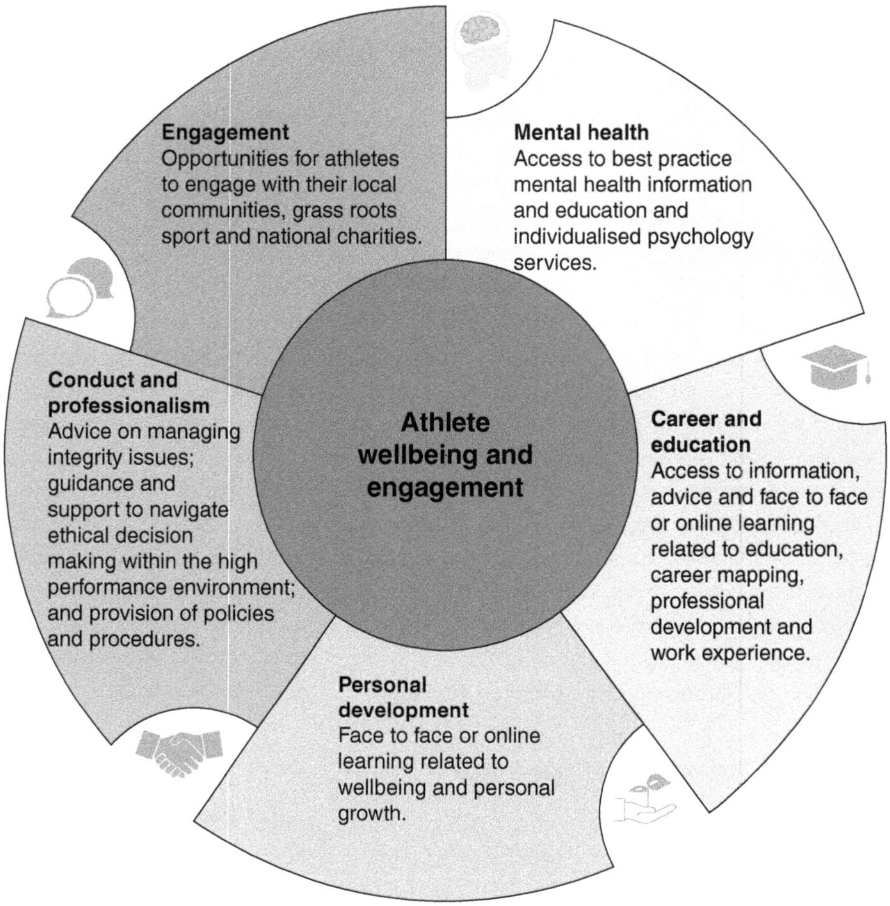

FIGURE 6.1 AIS Athlete Wellbeing and Engagement program: Five key domains of focus

Case: The Australian Institute of Sport (AIS) Mental Health Referral Network (MHRN)

The AIS MHRN provides eligible athletes and individuals from Australia's high performance sports system with priority access to a network of AIS approved service providers. These are comprised of psychologists, psychiatrists, and neuropsychologists across the country. The objective of the service is to ensure timely access to evidence-based intervention, provided by sufficiently skilled practitioners, in ways that meet the needs of elite athletes. The MHRN was conceived as an early intervention strategy, designed to yield better clinical outcomes for athletes, and in doing so, maximize the athlete's ability to reach their potential in their chosen sport. As previously noted, it was necessary to implement a decentralized model, given the organizational changes and move away from a centralized system at the AIS.

Orygen

Orygen's Elite Sport and Mental Health program was selected as an advisory partner and provided consultation to the AIS and Sport Australia regarding the procurement, commissioning and clinical governance model of the MHRN. Orygen was chosen in this capacity given the organization has played a major role in knowledge creation and dissemination for the youth mental health sector in Australia, and internationally (including via linkage with the World Economic Forum to develop a globally adaptable framework for youth mental health). Orygen also brings direct experience establishing nation-wide services for young people, where it founded the headspace early intervention model, funded federally throughout Australia and expanding globally (McGorry, Trethowan, & Rickwood, 2019; Rickwood et al., 2019), and in implementing processes to ensure model fidelity and assessment (Hetrick et al., 2018; Hughes et al., 2014).

Establishing the Mental Health Referral Network

The AIS MHRN commenced operation in late 2018, and is now actively supporting the mental health needs of athletes throughout Australia, and while they travel for sport internationally. In establishing the service, Sport Australia conducted procurement activities to establish a network of psychology service providers on a region-specific basis. In order to engage suitably qualified, experienced, and competent mental health professionals, the procurement process was targeted at practitioners recommended to the AIS from the National Institute Network, NSOs, lead psychologist and chief medical officer networks, in addition to athlete well-being and engagement managers. This phase targeted sole practitioners or heads of practices as individual private practitioners. Practitioners were required to have direct practical experience working within elite sports settings, or direct experience working with athlete populations, with demonstrated experience in the treatment of high prevalence disorders and psychosocial stressors among elite athletes (e.g., depression, anxiety, sleep difficulties, relationships, addictions, and exposure to trauma). All practitioners required a masters or doctoral level qualification in clinical psychology, or significant experience in sport and mental health (e.g., sports psychology). Once identified, practitioners were invited to submit an expression of interest covering several key criteria including their qualifications, experience and past performance in providing the required services, their capacity and availability to provide an accessible and responsive service, and the cost of their service. Their responses were assessed by a panel comprising the Mental Health Manager, an External Clinical Psychologist, and an additional AIS staff member with appropriate qualifications. When assessing potential psychiatrists against the AIS criteria, the panel also included an External Psychiatrist to ensure the panel had appropriate expertise.

The Mental Health Referral Network service

In the initial iteration of the MHRN, the service was established to provide support to the three highest levels of categorized athletes from both para and non-para sports (i.e., podium, podium ready, and podium potential classified athletes – those with a medal performance at the most recent world championship event and considered capable of a medal at the next world championship, or equivalent event). Referral to the MHRN could be made directly by athletes themselves, or by persons in the athlete's support network (e.g., family, sport staff). All referrals made to the MHRN are triaged by a Psychologist from the AIS Mental Health Team, comprising two registered Clinical Psychologists, a Clinical Psychology Registrar, and a Project Officer. This triage process determines the optimal mental health support strategy for the athlete. If the athlete is referred to a network service provider, the Mental Health Adviser forwards a Mental Health Referral Form, which includes key relevant information to the service provider to initiate a first consultation. Service provision occurs at the service provider's practice in one hour, face-to-face consultations with the athlete, unless circumstances require a non-face-to-face mode of consultation delivery (e.g., by telephone or online video consultation from the provider's practice). To ensure a timely response, the provider contacts the athlete within 24–48 hours to arrange the first appointment. Service providers are required to provide consultation with an athlete within two weeks for a standard referral and within one week for more urgent circumstances.

The MHRN service provider delivers appropriate evidence based treatment to the athlete for six initial consultation sessions. This is in line with the Australian Government's Better Access to Mental Health Care initiative, where government rebated mental health services are generally provided in a course of six treatment sessions initially. In some circumstances, delivery may need to be modified depending on athlete's needs, as discussed on a case-by-case basis. If more than six consultations sessions are required, the service provider seeks extension and approval from the Mental Health Manager of the Mental Health Team. In situations where additional case management support needs are identified, Mental Health Team staff, with permission from the athlete, will liaise with appropriate agencies to arrange such support. A summary of the timeline from referral to the MHRN to the end of service provision is outlined in Figure 6.2.

It is a requirement that MHRN practitioners provide evidence based treatments that are matched to the referred athlete's presenting problem. For example, evidence based treatments for affective and anxiety disorders (or symptoms) may include cognitive behavior therapy, behavioral activation, interpersonal therapy, rational emotive behavior therapy, problem solving therapy, or exposure response prevention. Other evidence based approaches may be applied as needed, including motivational interviewing for substance use problems and mindfulness or relaxation-based interventions (e.g., progressive muscle relaxation) for stress reduction.

To ensure athlete confidentiality, and in accordance with Australian standards (AHPRA, 2016), case file security and confidentiality remain the responsibility of the MHRN service provider. The AIS does not retain copies of the service provider's case file notes. So that the AIS can maintain program monitoring oversight, at the end of each month, the MHRN service provider is required to report de-identified data while ensuring they maintain athlete confidentiality and be within ethical guidelines for service providers. Information collected includes basic demographics (e.g., gender, age), primary reason for referral, number of sessions and referral pathway for further sessions (if required/desired). This information is used to identify the most frequent reasons for referral, emerging trends, and service demand, which then assists the AIS in developing broader early intervention initiatives and provides data to support future program resourcing.

In addition to the requirement for timely provision of the initial appointment, MHRN service providers need to ensure their availability for a minimum of six sessions following an athlete referral to their service. They are also required to attend network meetings and discussions and participate in any scheduled MHRN induction activities. MHRN service providers are further required to adhere to the AIS Mental Health Referral Network media policy (including social media), which is a mandated requirement of all AIS service providers, and to maintain an appropriate level of insurance, covering worker's compensation, public liability, and professional liability to meet the Federal Government requirements of agencies.

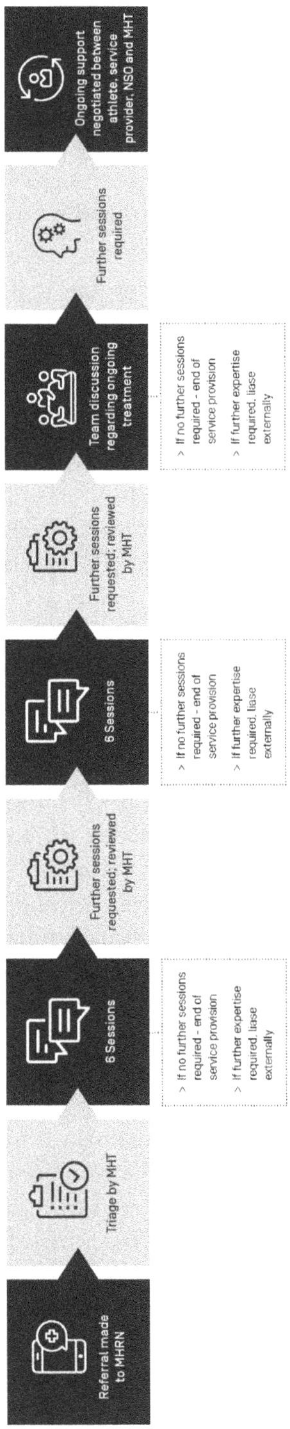

FIGURE 6.2 Mental Health Referral Network service provision timeline

Clinical governance

As a part of the development of the Mental Health Referral Network, the AIS, with advice from Orygen, reviewed best practice approaches to clinical governance in primary care and private mental health practice. A Clinical Governance Framework was then developed and implemented to ensure that there was clarity of relationships and responsibilities between the role of the AIS, the Mental Health Team, the MHRN service providers, and athletes as end users of the Network. It was critical to all that there was a robust framework in place to ensure that the network delivered safe and quality mental health care.

Reflections: Key lessons learned from the Mental Health Referral Network

Service delivery

Since commencing operation in late 2018, the AIS Mental Health Referral Network is now actively supporting the mental health needs of athletes throughout Australia, and has extended to servicing AIS athletes abroad, and to additional service providers, including psychiatry and neuropsychologists. At the time of writing, the AIS MHRN has received over 300 referrals, of which approximately 80% were referred on to a MHRN service provider. Almost all service providers have been able to arrange an initial appointment for the referred athlete within the required timeframes (two weeks for standard referrals, one week for more urgent referrals). In terms of treatment duration, the MHRN has been able to provide up to 12 consultation sessions per episode or care. In cases where referred athletes have required more than the initial six sessions approved by the Mental Health Team, an additional six sessions have been granted. If it became apparent that further sessions were required beyond those 12 sessions, a review was undertaken by the Mental Health Team in consultation with the service provider to clarify the anticipated number of extra consultation sessions needed based on clinical need. The Mental Health Team would evaluate this on a case-by-case basis according to clinical need and decide if this could continue to be provided within the MHRN at AIS cost. At the time of writing, the Mental Health Team were looking to implement evidence based decision-making processes to more systematically evaluate and respond to these requests.

Common presenting problems

Athletes referred to the MHRN presented with a range of problems, the most common being mild to moderate anxiety and depressive symptoms, which were impacting daily functioning. Other presenting or co-presenting problems included relationship difficulties, emotion regulation difficulties and stressful life events/exposure to traumatic events. A number of athletes also presented with sports-specific co-presenting issues, including injury, non-selection on the national team, and deselection from sport, social isolation when traveling, relationship difficulties within sport (e.g., with coaching staff or broader sporting organization), competing internationally in an individual sport, and retirement from sport. During the initial referral and triage process, the Mental Health Team worked hard to ensure that presenting issues were kept to those relating to mental health and psychosocial problems. This initial assessment was balanced with the need to provide accessibility of services to ensure athletes were receiving the support they required. Throughout this process, the Mental Health Team played a role in educating stakeholders (e.g., NSOs, National Institute Network [NIN]) on the types of presentations that were suitable for the service provision provided by the MHRN. This was particularly pertinent when considering presenting issues for athletes that might be relevant for the MHRN or that were more suitable to a performance psychology service (e.g., an athlete presenting with anxiety difficulties which were having a significant impact on their sports performance, but little to mild impact on other areas in their life). In differentiating the cases that arose, the Mental Health Team took the following approach for the acceptance of a referral; (i) the presenting difficulty was causing significant distress, (ii) the presenting difficulty impacted on daily functioning (another potential blurred boundary in that for many athletes, most of their time and daily routines occur within the daily training environment), and (iii) the presenting difficulty occurred in area(s) of life other than sports performance.

Adapting to the needs of the network: Changes made to service provision

An advantage that quickly emerged from the implementation of the MHRN was the opportunity it provided for a direct point of contact with the broader sports system, which allowed the Mental Health Team to develop a deeper level of knowledge about the system and provided an avenue to build trust with its key stakeholders. Building closer relationships between the AIS via the Mental Health Team and the NIN/NSOs has facilitated increased understanding and communication between these organizations, while providing an opportunity to receive feedback directly from stakeholders regarding the MHRN, and specifically what the mental health service needs of athletes are locally. The Mental Health Team has taken a flexible and responsive approach to adapting and evolving the MHRN, based on feedback received from stakeholders. A number of key learnings and adaptations have emerged, which have been considered and incorporated throughout the planning, rolling out, and consolidation phase of the MHRN, which we outline here.

A common tension that became evident during the initial phases of the MHRN was the decision for NIN/NSO's to manage mental health issues within the sport versus engaging outside expertise. In the past, there has been a tendency for sports to keep all matters 'in house', and this in part is thought to be due to concerns around maintaining confidentiality but also to ensure that key stakeholders within the sport (e.g., coaching staff) are across the concerns and problems being experienced by their individual athletes. This approach is often at odds with the preferences of the athlete, who anecdotally have in the past had a tendency to use an external service, particularly in the case of injury. The development of the MHRN responded to these contrasting preferences, through the development of a quality controlled external service that would allow athletes their autonomy but at the same time, build trust between the sports and external MHRN service providers to deliver services that are sensitive to the needs of the sport and the context in which they are being delivered (i.e., elite sporting context). To some degree, the success of gaining the sports trust and confidence in the MHRN is exemplified by the referral numbers made directly by the sports on the athlete's behalf, which has accounted for approximately half of the referrals received through the MHRN to date.

Another important change to the MHRN was that relating to the increased reach and scope of service delivery. In terms of reach, it quickly became evident that to fully meet the needs of the sports system, well-being services needed to stretch beyond the mental health service needs of top categorized athletes. Such expansion required greater resources, which were obtained, allowing the MHRN to expand service delivery to now service all categorized athletes, including developing and emerging athletes, as well as now providing services to high performance staff (e.g., coaches) and alumni (e.g., retired athletes requiring support with the transition out of sport). Additionally, in response to 'critical incidents' (e.g., sudden deaths within the high performance community, national disasters such as the 2019/2020 Australian bushfires, COVID-19), the MHRN has been able to further expand its available services to friends and family networks of those athletes and high performance staff directly impacted. In relation to increasing the scope of the service, other important learnings emerging from MHRN stakeholders was the need for further specialist services that emerged as being particularly relevant to the elite athlete population. For example, these specializations included having service providers with expertise in treating disordered eating and concussion. This has led to an increase in the type of service providers engaged by the Mental Health Team for MHRN service delivery, expanding beyond clinical psychologists to now include services provided by psychiatrists, neuropsychologists, psychologists with proven expertise in treating disordered Eating.

The MHRN is now in a consolidation phase where it is strengthening the services already being provided, as well as assessing how and where best to expand MHRN service provision. A number of key aspects have enabled this, one being the relationships developed with the sports system (e.g., NSOs, NIN), which has increased trust and communication and has provided the mechanism to receive 'real time' feedback from the sports network. The second being the AIS Mental Health Audit, the large, representative survey undertaken with AIS athletes, which is able to inform the service. Through these mechanisms, a number of areas for improvement and expansion have been identified, including improvements to the services catering for athletes from Paralympic sports. While these services are currently available, this is a target area for improvement for the MHRN. The Mental Health Team also sees a need for expansion in the conceptualization of service delivery and is motivated to move beyond service provision solely being reactive to illness but to instead take a more proactive and preventative approach to maximize and maintain well-being prior to the onset of more serious mental health problems.

Conclusions

The gains made by performance psychology and sports medicine over decades of research and practice serve as a motivating driver of what could be achieved in elite athlete mental health. Ultimately, however, programs that support athlete mental health transcend athletic achievement. They have the potential impact to support athletes to live meaningful lives regardless of their podium status. Such programs will likely improve career longevity and the ability of elite athletes to be inspirational ambassadors for their chosen sports. In this way, a program like the MHRN serves not just the aims of the athlete or sporting organization but may also have a positive impact on the broader culture around mental health and help-seeking behaviors.

References

AHPRA. (2016). Psychology board of Australia: Registration standard, from www.psychologyboard.gov.au/documents/default.aspx?record=WD16%2f19580&dbid=AP&chksum=NaZ6IJ8AQPuVCETcNMVDmg%3d%3d.

Arango, C., Díaz-Caneja, C. M., McGorry, P. D., Rapoport, J., Sommer, I. E., Vorstman, J. A., … Carpenter, W. (2018). Preventive strategies for mental health. *The Lancet Psychiatry 5*(7), 591–604. doi: 10.1016/S2215-0366(18)30057–9.

Goldberg, D. P., Gater, R., Sartorius, N., Ustun, T. B., Piccinelli, M., Gureje, O., & Rutter, C. (1997). The validity of two versions of the GHQ in the WHO study of mental illness in general health care. *Psychological Medicine 27*(1), 191–197. doi: 10.1017/S0033291796004242.

Hetrick, S. E., O'Connor, D. A., Stavely, H., Hughes, F., Pennell, K., Killackey, E., & McGorry, P. D. (2018). Development of an implementation guide to facilitate the roll-out of early intervention services for psychosis. *Early Interv Psychiatry 12*(6), 1100–1111. doi: 10.1111/eip.12420.

Hughes, F., Stavely, H., Simpson, R., Goldstone, S., Pennell, K., & McGorry, P. (2014). At the heart of an early psychosis centre: The core components of the 2014 Early Psychosis Prevention and Intervention Centre model for Australian communities. *Australas Psychiatry 22*(3), 228–234. doi: 10.1177/1039856214530479.

Markser, V. Z. (2011). Sport psychiatry and psychotherapy. Mental strains and disorders in professional sports. Challenge and answer to societal changes. *European Archives of Psychiatry and Clinical Neuroscience 261*, 182–185.

McGorry, P., Trethowan, J., & Rickwood, D. (2019). Creating headspace for integrated youth mental health care. *World Psychiatry 18*(2), 140–141. doi: 10.1002/wps.20619.

Orygen (2019). Retrieved from: www.orygen.org.au/About/News-And-Events/2019/Orygen-partners-with-World-Economic-Forum.

Purcell, R., Rice, S., Butterworth, M., & Clements, M. (2020). Rates and correlates of mental health symptoms in currently competing elite athletes from the Australian National High-Performance Sports System. *Sports Med*. doi: 10.1007/s40279-020-01266-z.

Reardon, C. L., Hainline, B., Aron, C. M., Baron, D., Baum, A. L., Bindra, A., … Engebretsen, L. (2019). Mental health in elite athletes: International Olympic Committee consensus statement (2019). *British Journal of Sports Medicine 53*(11), 667–699. doi: 10.1136/bjsports-2019–100715.

Rice, S. M., Parker, A. G., Rosenbaum, S., Bailey, A., Mawren, D., & Purcell, R. (2018). Sport-related concussion and mental health outcomes in elite athletes: A systematic review. *Sports Medicine 48*, 447–465.

Rice, S. M., Purcell, R., De Silva, S., Mawren, D., McGorry, P. D., & Parker, A. G. (2016). The mental health of elite athletes: A narrative systematic review. *Sports Medicine 46*, 1333–1353.

Rickwood, D., Paraskakis, M., Quin, D., Hobbs, N., Ryall, V., Trethowan, J., & McGorry, P. (2019). Australia's innovation in youth mental health care: The headspace centre model. *Early Intervention in Psychiatry 13*(1), 159–166. doi: 10.1111/eip.12740

Rosenberg, M. (1965). *Society and the adolescent self-image*. Princeton, NJ: Princeton University Press.

7

MENTAL HEALTH AND SPORT IN CANADA

An example of sport-focused collaborative care

Natalie Durand-Bush and Krista Van Slingerland

Context

Mounting evidence demonstrates that Canada's high-performance athletes experience mental health challenges and disorders; however, a number of barriers have prevented the holistic address of this population's mental health (Van Slingerland et al., 2019). For example, a lack of mental health policies and standardized best practices, low mental health literacy, stigmatizing cultural norms, and limited fragmented resource allocation have led to inconsistent mental health support across the Canadian high-performance sport system (Van Slingerland et al., 2019).

The development of a made-for-Canada mental health strategy for high-performance sport has been deemed necessary to inform and mobilize key stakeholders and organizations in the implementation of resources and services to promote mental health, prevent mental illness, and provide appropriate care to Canadian high-performance athletes experiencing mental health challenges. Consequently, an initiative to develop a Canadian national mental health strategy for high-performance sport was recently launched by Canadian sport leaders representing the Canadian Olympic and Paralympic Sport Institute Network (COPSIN), the Canadian Centre for Mental Health and Sport (CCMHS), Own the Podium (OTP), and Game Plan. While this group has begun to lay the groundwork for Canada's own address of mental health in high-performance sport, the strategy itself has not yet been finalized and implemented. This has arguably limited the availability and coordination of mental health care in Canadian high-performance sport to date, despite increasing demands. Nonetheless, an endeavor of this type and magnitude cannot be rushed. It is anticipated that the forthcoming strategy will fill an important gap in Canada's overall sport context.

The aim of this chapter is threefold. First, mental health in the Canadian high-performance sport context will be addressed through a foundational review of relevant mental health support pathways and organizations. Second, an example of sport-focused collaborative mental health care offered by the CCMHS, a novel national center dedicated to the mental health of Canadian athletes and coaches, will be provided. Third, recommendations to strengthen current mental health offerings and fulfill existing gaps within Canadian high-performance sport will be presented.

Mental health support pathways

To fully understand mental health in the Canadian sport context, it is important to provide an overview of mental health supports currently available to athletes both inside Canada's high-performance sport system (i.e., COPSIN and Game Plan), and outside of this system (i.e., CCMHS, Canadian Sport Psychology Association [CSPA], public and private health practitioners). Figure 7.1 provides a visual representation of the possible pathways to mental health care for Canadian athletes. It is evident that athletes have several options when seeking mental health care in Canada, which supports ethical and professional recommendations. Athletes must have choices and decide the best course of action according to their needs and preferences (e.g., work with practitioners within or outside the high-performance system). They must be able to provide free and informed consent to care at all times, which means they must agree of their own free will without pressure or threats and without altered faculties, and they must receive all the information required to make a decision with full knowledge of the facts (i.e., nature and purpose of care, anticipated effects, procedures to be used, possible risks, possible side effects, other possible mental health care options, probable impact on health and well-being if they refuse care). This implies that athletes are aware of all of their options when seeking mental health care, however, this is not always the case. Consequently, sport stakeholders and practitioners have an important role to play in this process to ensure that athletes can make informed decisions with regards to their own mental health care. Following is an overview of athletes' possible pathways to care in Canada.

COPSIN referral pathway. COPSIN provides world-leading training environments to elite athletes and coaches across Canada. The team of experts delivers sport science and medicine, coaching, research and innovation, education and Game Plan services to power podium performances and help Canada win more medals. The Network includes four Canadian Sport Institutes (Pacific, Calgary, Ontario, and Québec) and three Canadian Sport Centers (Saskatchewan, Manitoba, and Atlantic). Athletes who are registered members of a Canadian Sport Institute (CSI) or a Canadian Sport Centre (CSC) can access mental health support through their Institute/Centre's Mental Performance Lead (MPL) or Game Plan Advisor. Athletes may self-identify as needing support, or may be flagged by their coach, or a member of their integrated support team. Some CSIs screen for mental health challenges and may identify athletes who are struggling via this mechanism; however, most CSI/CSCs do not take this proactive approach.

Once athletes are identified, they are directed to appropriate resources. This may be their MPL, who may provide them with support if they are trained to do so, or the MPL will refer to internal or external practitioners (e.g., psychologist, psychotherapist, counsellor, psychiatrist, specialized clinic, Morneau Shepell). Access to funding to subsidize care varies across CSI/Cs, so athletes may be able to receive support free of charge (via in-house services) or may have support up to a limited number of sessions (e.g., ~5 sessions) or dollar amount (e.g., up to $500/athlete per year). While athletes have access to the Canadian Athlete Insurance Program (CAIP), this only provides support for accidental and overuse injuries sustained in sport. While the CAIP does provide some coverage for "psychological therapy," the therapy must be necessary due to an accidental or overuse injury. Importantly, mental health challenges and disorders are not considered an injury under the Policy's terms and conditions, which is an unfortunate limitation of this program.

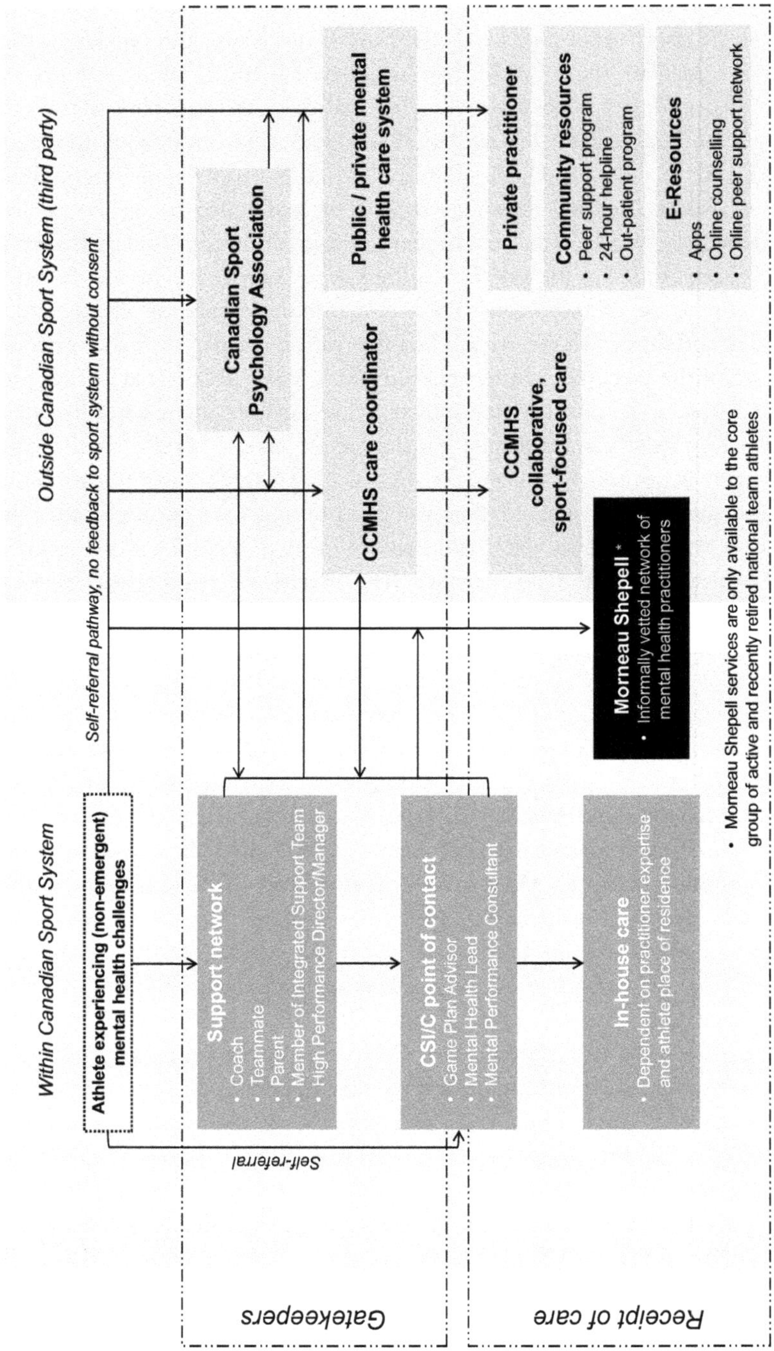

FIGURE 7.1 Possible pathways to mental health care for Canadian athletes

Game Plan. Game Plan is a total athlete wellness program that supports Canadian senior national team athletes across their high-performance career and as they transition out of sport. Sport Canada carded athletes – or national training group athletes deemed by their National Sport Organization (NSO) to be at the senior national team level – in a Paralympic, Olympic, Pan Am, or Para Pan Am discipline, have full access to Game Plan services. Game Plan offers eligible athletes a number of resources and opportunities related to employment, networking, education, skill development, and health and wellness. Through Game Plan's partner Morneau Shepell, athletes have access to a range of services including mental health support accessible via live chat, phone, or email. Once registered with Game Plan, athletes may access mental health support themselves (i.e., self-refer), or receive support from their CSI/CSC, Game Plan Advisor, or allied health practitioner (e.g., external Mental Performance Consultant [MPC], sport medicine physician) to navigate the system. Through the partnership, Morneau Shepell covers the cost of eight sessions with a Morneau Shepell mental health practitioner. Athletes can also get financial assistance and obtain at least $500 through the COPSI Network. It is worth mentioning that most Morneau Shepell practitioners are not trained in high-performance sport, which may impact the therapeutic alliance developed with athletes and limit the outcomes of therapy. Anecdotal feedback gathered by Game Plan shows that this is the case roughly 50% of the time. Athletes returning to their MPL or Game Plan advisor after unsuccessful interactions with any practitioner will be directed to another one until there is an appropriate fit.

Canadian Centre for Mental Health and Sport (CCMHS). The CCMHS is a registered charity supporting the mental health and performance of competitive and high-performance athletes and coaches. The CCMHS offers collaborative, *sport-focused* mental health care services designed to help competitive and high-performance athletes and coaches achieve their performance goals while preserving their mental health and well-being. Uniquely, all CCMHS practitioners (i.e., psychologists, counsellors, psychotherapists, MPCs, psychiatrist, physician) have training or a background in high-performance sport, and care is delivered in person and/or via telehealth technology. To be eligible for CCMHS services, athletes or coaches must be 16 years of age or older, competing at the provincial level or higher, and be experiencing clinical symptoms that cause impairments to their functioning in sport. Approximately half of CCMHS service-users presently receiving care are current or former national team athletes.

The CCMHS operates on a fee-for-service basis. While the Centre covers the cost of athletes or coaches' first session (intake), the remaining cost of care are incurred by the service-user, which can be prohibitive for some athletes and coaches. For those who have coverage through private insurance, the care plan is optimized to take advantage of this. The D'Arcy Bush Memorial Fund provides the CCMHS with some ability to subsidize sessions for athletes and coaches who cannot afford the cost of care.

Mental Performance Consultants (MPCs) / Canadian Sport Psychology Association (CSPA). MPCs working in high-performance sport in Canada are typically registered professional members with the Canadian Sport Psychology Association (CSPA). The CSPA is an "applied sport psychology organization aiming to facilitate the development of mental and emotional skills, attitudes, perspectives, strategies, and processes that lead to optimal performance, well-being, and personal growth" (CSPA, 2020). It has as a mandate to evaluate and list MPCs who meet minimum requirements to provide mental performance services in Canada, and recognize those working as licensed or registered psychologists. Only a handful have this dual MPC / psychologist credential up to date (CSPA, 2020). At a minimum, MPCs hold a master's and/

or doctoral degree in sport psychology or a related field. They have knowledge and skills in sport sciences, psychology, and counseling, and provide individual and/or group consultations geared toward improving sport performance and overall functioning and well-being. Unless they have received the same training as that of psychologists or psychotherapists, they do not diagnose and treat mental health problems.

MPCs are in an ideal position to recognize and respond to athletes who are struggling with their mental health. MPCs may be the trusted individuals to whom athletes disclose their challenges. In other cases, they may be the ones within athletes' integrated support teams noting significant shifts in their behaviors, appearance, and overall functioning, suggesting that they may be in need of additional support. While few NSOs employ MPCs on a full or part-time basis, many of them will contract MPCs to provide services to athletes in preparation for major games or competitions. Athletes may choose to work with MPCs within or outside the formal high-performance sport network; however, the costs of services are typically incurred by the athletes. MPCs who have to refer athletes to mental health practitioners when issues are beyond their scope of practice can do so by accessing professionals within or outside the high-performance system, depending on the availability and accessibility of services and resources.

Public/private mental health care. While there are several advantages to working with mental health practitioners within the existing sport system (e.g., established relationships, communication, and coordination of services), some athletes will opt to seek external third-party services in which confidentiality is fully safeguarded and there are no political and organizational influences or biases. Examples of "at arm's length" services include not only the CCMHS but also traditional public/private mental health care. Psychiatric services are covered by *public* health insurance in Canada and athletes requiring medication for a mental illness are often directed to a psychiatrist. Services rendered by a psychologist, counsellor, or psychotherapist on the other hand, are not covered by public health insurance, but *private* health insurance may cover all or some of these services. Athletes can also access other public/private mental health services and resources, including anonymous and self-directed interventions online (e.g., apps, toll-free helpline, e-counseling) and in the community (e.g., peer-support network).

In sum, Canadians in high-performance sport acknowledge that mental health challenges require attention, although funding for adequate, longitudinal supports remains a major constraint. At the moment, there are several pathways within and outside the high-performance sport system available to athletes for mental health care, and there are advantages and disadvantages to each pathway. A Canadian national mental health strategy for high-performance sport is currently under development. It is anticipated that this strategy will be vital in informing, mobilizing, and coordinating Canadian stakeholders in their efforts to promote mental health, prevent mental illness, and offer mental health care for those experiencing mental illness.

Case

The following case focuses on one particular organization in Canada specializing in the provision of mental health care for high-performance athletes and coaches, that is, the CCMHS. The CCMHS was launched in September 2018 following an evidence-informed process in which sport and mental health stakeholders collaborated to design a *sport-focused* mental health care model and national center, which became the CCMHS (Van Slingerland, Durand-Bush, & Kenttä, 2020). There are several unique features to the CCMHS. Specifically, in comparison to traditional mental health care options that are currently available in Canada, the

CCMHS offers value-added services that are captured by its 4Cs features (i.e., sport-Centered, Comprehensive, Collaborative, and Convenient), which are explained next.

sport-Centered

With regards to its sport-Centered focus, CCMHS practitioners have training in counseling, psychology, and sport sciences. They understand the intricacies of the competitive sport environment, and have extensive experience working with competitive and high-performance athletes and coaches. Many of them were competitive athletes and/or coaches themselves, and are now parents of competitive athletes. This knowledge and experience allows them to tailor therapeutic approaches based on relevant sport-specific factors (e.g., performance demands, competitive pressure, sport specialization, year-round training/coaching, coaching style, funding, injuries, transitions in and out of sport, peak and recovery periods, diet restrictions, team members, sport culture, traveling schedule, anti-doping regulations). As a result, practitioners are able to establish strong and credible therapeutic alliances with athlete and coach clients, and provide accurate diagnoses and recommendations when treating mental illnesses and improving mental health and mental performance. This has been deemed important by several researchers and practitioners working in high-performance sport (Henriksen et al., 2020; Reardon et al., 2019; Van Slingerland et al., 2019).

Collaborative

Another feature is that CCMHS practitioners work as an integrated unit and collaborate on a regular basis to determine and adjust care plans. Of note, the CCMHS team includes practitioners representing all core mental health and mental performance regulated professions in Canada (e.g., counsellors, psychotherapists, psychologists, psychiatrists, MPCs). Practitioners also work with clients' extended support team, as permitted by the clients, to optimize care as well and transitions in and out of the CCMHS. For example, they can discuss care plans with existing team physicians for additional support while athletes are away at a competition. This allows continuity of care and decreases contradictory recommendations that could negatively impact sport performance (e.g., psychiatrist recommends a break from sport until medication is stabilized while on-site team physician suggests only reducing number of hours of training). See Figure 7.2 for an overview of the CCMHS collaborative care model. It is important to note that all CCMHS clients provide informed consent to receive collaborative care by the core mental health care team. A distinct process is followed to obtain clients' consent to share any information with the extended mental health care team and their referral and support network.

Collaborative models of care have been recognized as the gold standard to effectively address mental health and addiction issues (Gregory, 2009; Kates et al., 2011). In their case study of an elite athlete receiving care from the CCMHS, Van Slingerland, Durand-Bush, DesClouds, et al. (2020) reported that "among other advantages, collaborative models leverage the strengths and differences of multidisciplinary practitioners within an individual's circle of care to provide the most comprehensive support available" (p. 18).

Of importance is the flexibility of the collaboration that can occur between CCMHS practitioners. At a minimum, two practitioners (i.e., a Lead and a Support) are assigned to each client's Collaborative Care Team (CCT). This helps to ensure that a practitioner is available

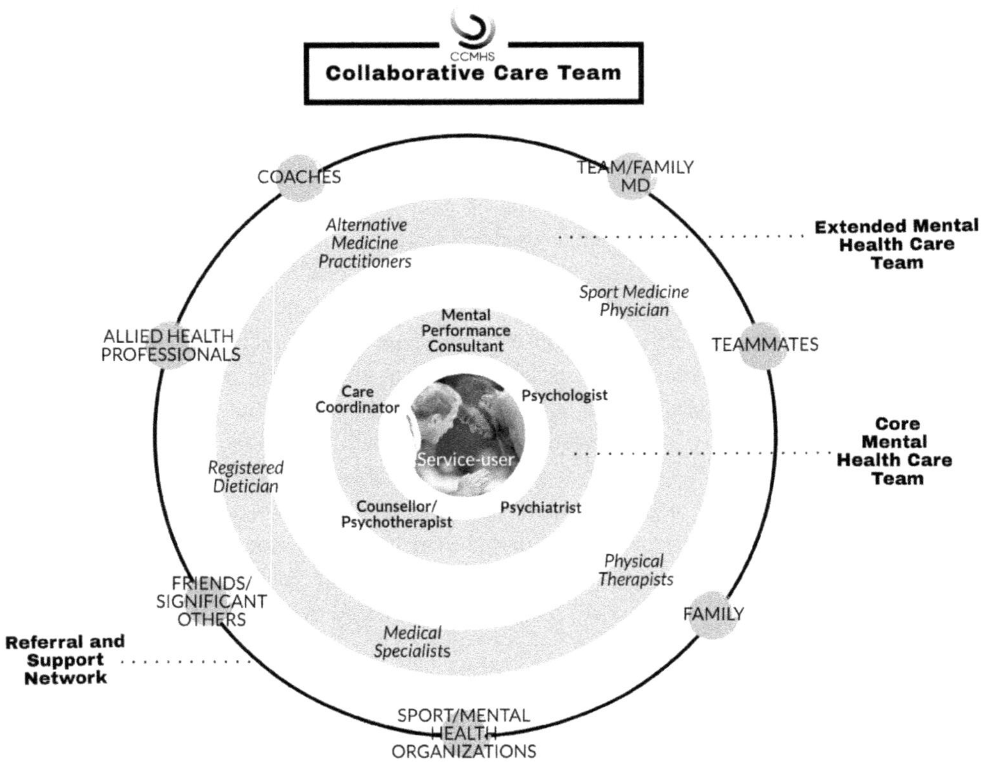

FIGURE 7.2 CCMHS collaborative care model

should an urgent matter arise, specific needs are addressed by whichever CCT member is most appropriate (based on area(s) of specialization), different time-zones are accommodated, provincial restrictions regarding care provision (e.g., psychologists must be registered in the province in which their client resides) are respected, and a culture of learning and professional development amongst practitioners is fostered (Van Slingerland, Durand-Bush, DesClouds, et al., 2020).

As depicted in Jones and Way's (2006) model (see Figure 7.3), collaborative care within the CCMHS varies from independent parallel practice, to consultation/referral, to interdependent co-provision of care, depending on the complexity of the case, the availability and areas of specialization of practitioners forming the CCT, and the geographical location of both clients and practitioners. For example, practitioners can work independently if they do not perceive a need for additional input and support. This is not uncommon given the dual mental health and mental performance competencies that practitioners have. In other cases, practitioners within a CCT will consult with one another to get insight into a proposed course of action (e.g., refrain from competing in an upcoming competition) or to resolve a particular issue (e.g., telehealth challenge). They may also refer a client to another practitioner on the team who conducts specialized assessments (e.g., ADHD) or uses a particular therapeutic approach or technique (e.g., bio-neurofeedback). Finally, some practitioners within a CCT will work together throughout the provision of care given the complexity of a case (e.g., comorbidities, suicidal ideation) and geographical location (e.g., psychologist works in person with the client

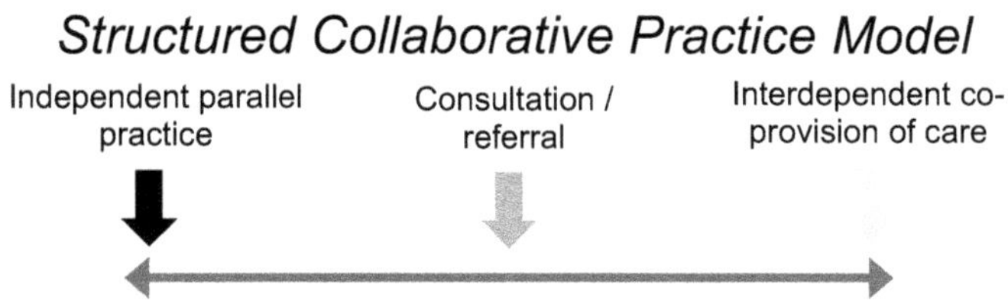

FIGURE 7.3 Collaborative practice model

to discuss mental health issues while the MPC conducts sessions via the telehealth platform to work on resilience training).

Comprehensive

As can be seen in the previous section, CCMHS practitioners aim to put in place specific and relevant care plans that take into account the complex roles, identities, and demands that athletes or coaches must manage within their sport system and culture throughout a competitive season and quadrennium (e.g., plans respect training and competition standards, goals, and schedules, and address coach/teammates/family/support staff demands). This is vital given that within gifted or talented populations (i.e., elite athletes), perceptions that practitioners lack an in-depth understanding of the specialized characteristics and environmental demands of a particular domain is a significant deterrent to help-seeking (Levy & Plucker, 2003). Indeed, being familiar with or having competed in sport was athletes' number one preferred quality in a counselor according to Lopez and Levy (2013). Failing to put in place specialized treatment plans that meticulously address the demands, pressures, and adversity that athletes or coaches must manage within their sport can jeopardize the effectiveness of care and sustainability of therapeutic outcomes (Henriksen et al., 2020).

Convenient

Athletes and coaches in high-performance sport have demanding schedules and extensive travel commitments throughout a competitive season and Olympic/Paralympic quadrennium (Henriksen et al., 2020). As such, mental health care must be provided in a timely, efficient, and reliable manner. CCMHS practitioners follow a systematic and speedy process spanning the intake (i.e., assessment of eligibility criteria and needs), referral to a CCT, provision of mental health care, and exit from the CCMHS (see Van Slingerland, Durand-Bush, DesClouds, et al., 2020 for a specific example). Practitioners are flexible and accommodating to best meet the needs and preferences of clients (e.g., offer extended hours of services throughout the week and weekend, with on-call practitioners for emergencies). Practitioners also provide both in-person and telehealth services to accommodate clients' various sport contexts (e.g., training outside of the country) as well as schedule and travel constraints (e.g., work remotely as needed). On average, it takes 11 days (including weekends) from the time clients complete an intake with the CCMHS Care Coordinator to the time their CCT is assigned and they are ready to begin therapy. This is remarkable given that Canadians can wait up to a year to receive mental health support through Canada's traditional health system (Canadian Mental Health Association, 2017).

In sum, this case gives a glimpse into the specialized mental health care offered by the CCMHS. As the first national center in Canada to provide collaborative sport-focused services to athletes and coaches, it is clear that specific and contextualized knowledge and training in high-performance sport facilitates the provision of mental health care, which encompasses diagnosis, treatment, monitoring, and recovery. The CCMHS is an important pathway that relies on evidence-based approaches and a comprehensive team of specialists to prioritize both mental health and athletic performance in its education and mental health care initiatives.

Reflections

In light of the information provided in this chapter, including existing mental health pathways and organizations, as well as the literature in the area of mental health and sport, a number of recommendations are offered to strengthen current mental health offerings and fulfill remaining gaps in Canada's high-performance sport system.

Psycho-education

To date, there is no systematic provision of mental health education to high-performance athletes, coaches, and support staff. The psychoeducational tools that have been developed by organizations such as Game Plan and the CCMHS are not consistently available in a permanent online location and may not be accessible to athletes at the lower levels of the talent identification pathway. These are missed opportunities for early education and intervention, particularly at the Next Gen and Development levels of the Canadian sport system. Thus, democratizing these resources is a cost-effective way for improving the accessibility and reach of trainings, and increasing mental health literacy across the sport system.

Mental health screening

Preventative mental health screening protocols are not consistently in place across Canada's high-performance sport system. Enacting standardized protocols would assist in identifying mental health challenges *early,* positioning mental health as a core component of optimal sport performance, and destigmatizing mental health challenges within the Canadian sport community. Standardized screening protocols would also remove barriers to help seeking (i.e., stigma, lack of self-awareness) by eliminating the need for athletes to self-identify as struggling.

Prevention and management through planning

Mental health challenges and crises may occur despite best efforts to provide resources that promote and protect mental health in high-performance sport. Planning for the prevention and management of challenges or crises takes some of the uncertainty out of high-stress and highly nuanced situations. Presently, many NSOs are not taking a proactive approach to plan for mental health challenges and crises. A mental health action plan is a plug-and-play guide for athletes to complete and discuss with their coach, MPC, Game Plan advisor, and/or high-performance director. A preventative tool, the mental health action plan prompts athletes to reflect on what they need from coaches and others (e.g., IST members, parents) to feel supported and best perform in training and competition – both when they are well, *and* when they are experiencing mental health challenges. By setting expectations, managing mental health challenges and crises becomes part of team culture and norms, and are therefore received more favorably by those surrounding athletes who are struggling.

Signposting

The Canadian high-performance sport system lacks clear and coordinated "signposting" through which established referral pathways to mental health support available to athletes, coaches, and support staff are communicated. Signposting empowers those seeking support and encourages efficient use of resources by helping individuals navigate complex health systems to find the most appropriate source of support. From an ethical standpoint, all available pathways to mental health care should be articulated to high-performance sport athletes so they may select the most suitable option for them.

Confidentiality

Within current pathways to subsidized care in high-performance sport, there is little opportunity for athletes to receive financial support without reporting that they are accessing care to funders (i.e., NSO, CSI/CSC, Game Plan). Research shows that athletes are reluctant to seek help because they fear their coaches and teammates will find out (Gulliver, Griffiths, & Christensen, 2012). The ability to self-refer in a confidential manner is vital as it facilitates help-seeking and may encourage more frequent and earlier help-seeking among athletes.

Care subsidization

The average number of mental health care sessions currently subsidized by members of the COPSIN (~4) does not meet clinically suggested threshold for facilitating optimal recovery from mental health challenges and disorders (e.g., 6–8 sessions for depression; Forde et al., 2005). As such, it is possible that athletes are not returning to optimal health before returning to play. Additional funding is required to ensure that athletes receive adequate longitudinal care.

Return to play protocols

The majority of organizations (i.e., NSOs, CSCs/CSIs) have not established protocols and procedures for re-integrating athletes into training and competition following mental health challenges or crises that take them out of play. Such processes are particularly important in team sports, where a culture of accountability to more than oneself creates social pressure to meet team standards and expected behaviors. While each case is highly individualized, broad protocols that indicate the steps to return to training and competition, including who can clear athletes to resume activity, and at what level, will limit ambiguity and set expectations for all parties involved.

Stay in play

Every individual's experience of mental health challenges and disorders is unique. While for some disorders (e.g., eating disorders, burnout, manic phase of bipolar disorder), it is not safe to continue training and competing until symptoms are managed or stabilized, many athletes (e.g., those suffering from mild to moderate anxiety or depression) are able to compete while managing symptoms of mental illness. The development of guidelines or best practices for the management of mental health challenges while staying in sport would support the implementation of measures (e.g., reduced training load) to assist athletes in safely training and competing while working toward recovery.

Coach well-being

Despite research indicating that coaches are particularly susceptible to mental health challenges such as burnout (McNeil, Durand-Bush, & Lemyre, 2016), limited mental health support is provided to coaches within the high-performance sport system. It is concerning that there is no established duty of care owed by organizations to coaching staff when it comes to mental health. Evidence suggests that mentally healthy coaches create healthier environments for their athletes (Stebbings, Taylor, & Spray, 2011). Thus, caring for coaches can be regarded as a preventative measure against debilitative actions known to occur within the coach-athlete dyad (e.g., controlling coaching style, maltreatment) that can compromise athletes' mental health.

Interprovincial regulations and telehealth

Interprovincial practice regulations prohibit psychologists and psychiatrists from providing long-term support to athletes who are not residents of the province or territory in which they are licensed to practice. This is significant because many athletes will relocate to different areas of the country to train. The use of telehealth technology is growing and offers flexibility when providing care to migratory athletes. However, mental health practitioners report that individuals with complex challenges (e.g., co-morbid disorders) should be seen in person. Consequently, pathways for mental health care in high-performance sport should incorporate both in-person and telehealth options. Further, given the unique needs of the athletic population, the development of national in-person and telehealth regulations permitting the provision of care across provincial and territorial borders is necessary.

In sum, mental health is a priority and responsibility that must be shared by every stakeholder in high-performance sport. A collaborative and coordinated national strategy is necessary to protect and promote mental health and prevent and manage mental illness in athletes, coaches, and support staff. Regardless of best practices and efforts, many individuals will experience mental health challenges and disorders. The Canadian high-performance sport system currently benefits from the support of multiple mental health care pathways and organizations. However, if the goal is to build, optimize, and preserve mental health in this country, there is room for improvement and growth.

References

Canadian Mental Health Association. (2017, May 5). *Wait times*. Canadian Mental Health Association. https://cmha.ca/wait-times-2

Canadian Sport Psychology Association. (2020). *About*. Available at: www.cspa-acps.com/about

Forde, F., Frame, M., Hanlon, P., MacLean, G., Nolan, D., Shajahan, P., & Troy, E. (2005). Optimum number of sessions for depression and anxiety. *Nursing Times 101*(43), 36–40.

Gregory, S. (2009). Collaborative care for mood disorders. *Current Opinion in Psychiatry 22*(1), 37–41. doi:10.1097/YCO.0b013e328313e3f0.

Gulliver, A., Griffiths, K. H., & Christensen, H. (2012). Barriers and facilitators to mental health help-seeking for young elite athletes: A qualitative study. *BMC Psychiatry 12*, 157. https://doi.org/10.1186/1471-244X-12–157.

Jones, L., & Way, D. (2006). *Collaborative practice learning guide.* Ottawa, ON: Supporting Interdisciplinary Practice.

Henriksen, K., Schinke, R., McCann, S., Durand-Bush, N., Moesch, K., Parham, W. D., … Hunziker, J. (2020). Athlete mental health in the Olympic/Paralympic quadrennium: A multi-societal consensus statement. *International Journal of Sport and Exercise Psychology.* https://doi.org/10.1080/1612197X.2020.1746379.

Kates, N., Mazowita, G., Lemire, F., Jayabarathan, A., Bland, R., Selby, P., … Audet, D. (2011). The evolution of collaborative mental health care in Canada: A shared vision for the future. *The Canadian Journal of Psychiatry 56*(5), 1–5.

Levy, J. J., & Plucker, J. A. (2003). Assessing the psychological presentation of gifted and talented clients: A multicultural perspective. *Counselling Psychology Quarterly 16,* 229–247. https://psycnet.apa.org/doi/10.1080/0951507031000161010O.

Lopez, R., & Levy, J. (2013). Student athletes' perceived barriers to and preferences for seeking counseling. *Journal of College Counseling 16*(1), 19–31. https://doi.org/10.1002/j.2161-1882.2013.00024.x.

McNeill, K., Durand-Bush, N., & Lemyre, P-N. (2016). Understanding coach burnout and underlying emotions: A narrative approach. *Sports Coaching Review 5*(1), 1–18. https://doi.org/10.1080/21640629.2016.1163008.

Reardon, C., Hainline, B., Miller Aron, C., Baron, D., Baum, A. L., Bindra, A., … Engebretsen, L. (2019). Mental health in elite athletes: International Olympic Committee consensus statement (2019). *British Journal of Sports Medicine 53,* 667–699. http://dx.doi.org/10.1136/bjsports-2019-100715.

Stebbings, J., Taylor, I. M., & Spray, C. M. (2011). Antecedents of perceived coach autonomy supportive and controlling behaviors: Coach psychological need satisfaction and well-being. *Journal of Sport & Exercise Psychology, 33,* 255–272. https://doi.org/10.1123/jsep.33.2.255.

Van Slingerland, K. J., Durand-Bush, N., Bradley, L., Goldfield, G., Archambault, R., Smith, D., … Kenttä, G. (2019). Canadian Centre for Mental Health and Sport (CCMHS) position statement: Principles of mental health in competitive and high-performance sport. *Clinical Journal of Sport Medicine 29,* 173–180. http://dx.doi.org/10.1097/JSM.0000000000000665.

Van Slingerland, K. J., Durand-Bush, N., DesClouds, P., & Kenttä, G. (2020). Providing mental health care to an elite athlete: The perspective of the Canadian Centre for Mental Health and Sport (CCMHS) team. *Case Studies in Sport and Exercise Psychology 4,* S1-17–S1-26. https://doi.org/10.1123/cssep.2019-0022.

Van Slingerland, K. J., Durand-Bush, N., & Kenttä, G. (2020). Collaboratively designing the Canadian Centre for Mental Health and Sport (CCMHS) using group concept mapping. *Journal of Applied Sport Psychology 33*(1), 98–122. https://doi.org/10.1080/10413200.2019.1704938.

PART II

Specific interventions on mental health across countries

8

ACT FOR HEALTH ANXIETY AND PERFORMANCE READINESS

Alexander Cohen

Context

The USOPC is focused on protecting, supporting and empowering America's athletes, and is responsible for fielding US teams for the Olympic, Paralympic, Youth Olympic, Pan American and Parapan American Games, and serving as the steward of the Olympic and Paralympic movements in the United States. Our mission is to "Empower Team USA athletes to achieve sustained competitive excellence and well-being."

To help achieve this mission, the USOPC employs several full time Sport Psychologists who provide sport psychology consultation for national teams, athletes, and coaches at the Olympic and Paralympic Training Centers, at National Governing Body training sites, and at national and international competitions. As licensed psychologists with expertise in the psychology of performance excellence, we work within multiple interdisciplinary teams, frequently collaborating with sports medicine, sports nutrition, strength and conditioning, physiology, coaching education, and other mental health and sport psychology professionals.

As a USOPC Senior Sport Psychologist, I assist coaches in creating supportive performance environments that promote psychological and physical skill acquisition and mastery. I work directly with athletes to maximize performance readiness through consistent preparation, enhanced resilience, and mindful self-regulation.

Though initially trained from a Cognitive-Behavioral Therapy (CBT) perspective toward sport psychology and counseling psychology, my practice is more recently influenced by Acceptance and Commitment Therapy, one of the "third wave" behavioral therapies. ACT (pronounced as the word "act") is a mindfulness-based behavioral therapy grounded on the philosophy of Functional Contextualism and Relational Frame Theory (Hayes, Strosahl, & Wilson, 2012). Created in 1986 by Steve Hayes, ACT utilizes an eclectic mix of metaphor, paradox, and mindfulness skills, along with a wide range of experiential exercises and values-guided behavioral interventions. As Harris (2006) states, the goal of ACT is to create a rich and meaningful life, while accepting the pain that inevitably goes with it. "ACT is about taking effective action guided by our deepest values and in which we are fully present and engaged. It is only through mindful action that we can create a meaningful life" (Harris, 2006, p. 2).

Sport psychologists are typically fond of encouraging athletes to "focus on the process," which aligns nicely with the ACT approach of being fully engaged in the present moment. As such, I have found ACT to be an excellent framework for facilitating athlete *Performance Readiness*, which I define as the ability to focus on the right thing, at the right time, every time. While this is certainly aspirational, I have found that athletes enjoy being challenged to focus as consistently as possible. While results are rarely entirely under an athlete's control, the ability to focus under pressure is. This means that athletes can view competition in terms of "who aims their attention the best" rather than being exclusively based on physical prowess. Focusing on the "right" thing at the "right" time is to be interpreted in the Buddhist sense of "rightness" as in the Noble Eightfold Path (NEP; Nilsson & Kazemi, 2016a; Olendzki, 2013). The NEP provides the ethical context for development and serves as guidelines for living life and being in the present moment. It consists of: (a) right view, (b) right intention, (c) right speech, (d) right action, (e) right livelihood, (f) right effort, (g) right mindfulness, (h) right concentration. The NEP is further divided into three major parts: (a) concentration (right effort, right mindfulness, right concentration), (b) wisdom (right view, right intention), and (c) ethical conduct (right speech, right action, right livelihood). It is important to recognize that "right" in the NEP is not meant to signify rigid, normative behavior. Rather, it is a sense of being well-tuned and able to discern wholesome from unwholesome actions (Nilsson & Kazemi, 2016a; Olendzki, 2013). Similarly, in the context of performance readiness, "rightness" refers to being and acting with skilfulness and intentionality, as consistently as possible (i.e., "every time"). Focusing on the right thing, at the right time, every time is therefore a commitment to moving in a valued direction (Harris, 2009). Performance readiness is a value that serves to guide action, rather than an expectation that one will focus perfectly in all situations. It is a way for athletes to translate their values into committed action during training and competition. Psychological flexibility is inherent in this approach, as athletes are encouraged to hold this value lightly, but pursue it vigorously (Harris, 2011).

ACT has been adapted for many presenting issues, one of which is health anxiety. As noted by Eilenberg, Frostholm, and Kronstrand (2014), health anxiety causes great personal suffering, places a substantial burden on health services and treatment is an important challenge to health care providers. Health anxiety is characterized by exaggerated rumination with intrusive worries about harboring serious illness and a persistent preoccupation with one's health leading to significant impairment and a decrease in quality of life.

The following case study demonstrates the application of ACT with an elite female endurance athlete experiencing health anxiety. My hope is that this case illustrates the versatility of ACT in addressing this type of complex issue while simultaneously facilitating greater performance readiness in training and competition.

Case

When presenting a case study, a balance must be sought between providing useful information and preserving athlete confidentiality. To minimize the risk of identification, the athlete's name and sport, reference to geographical locations, and other personal details have been changed or omitted.

The athlete is a 20-year-old endurance athlete competing at the National Team level in her sport. Her long-term goals include graduating from college and being an Olympic medalist. For confidentiality, I will refer to her as "Jane."

Jane was referred to me by her coaches and her team's sports medicine professionals to explore her health concerns that were interfering with training and competition. She presented as an engaging, determined athlete. Frequently smiling, she came across as positive, introspective, and open to support. While Jane's team engaged in weekly mindfulness meditation sessions, Jane had not previously worked individually with a sport psychologist or mental health therapist.

After discussing her concerns, Jane and I agreed to approach this as a case of health anxiety. We continued collaborating with her medical team to evaluate potential issues that might underly her symptom presentation. Jane also stated that a goal in working with me would be to "stop overthinking things and be ok with things not always going as planned." She noted that she "really wanted to try to worry less about issues that are not very important, just to let things go sometimes" and that she wanted to "race at the highest level and do everything possible to be the best that I can be."

Jane stated that one of her parents passed away unexpectedly when she was younger, and that she had good relationships with her surviving parent and sibling. She stated that she had several "amazing friends" inside and outside of her sport and had "super great teammates and coaches."

When asked about her strengths as a person and performer, she stated, "I am pretty good at pushing myself really hard. I also feel like I'm good at managing pre-race nerves and channeling them into energy. As a person, I think I am good at working hard and putting a lot in to the things that I am passionate about."

Jane experienced rumination with intrusive worries about the presence of possible illness. She stated that the preoccupation with her health led to disruptions in training and competition and somewhat affected her overall quality of life. In her words, "The main way that it affects other areas of my life is that I sometimes am just super preoccupied with a minor health issue or any abnormality that I notice, which can affect my focus."

When queried about any changes or significant events that may have coincided with the start of her health anxiety, Jane stated, "I got pretty sick for a while and just couldn't get rid of a lot of the symptoms." She described experiencing fatigue, occasional heart arrhythmias ("it's as if my heart skips a beat"), weakness, stomach pain, headaches, shortness of breath, and gastrointestinal symptoms, all of which were quite disruptive for an endurance athlete.

The preceding description of symptoms brings us to an important point about ACT and health anxiety. Harris (2006) notes that in stark contrast to most Western psychotherapy, ACT does not have symptom reduction as a goal. Jane described the physical sensations she was experiencing as "symptoms," and also shared the thoughts and feelings ("private experiences") that accompanied these sensations. The distinction between symptoms, physical sensations, and the thoughts, feelings, and perceptions about these physical sensations is important. Harris (2006) states:

> As soon as a private experience is labelled a "symptom", it immediately sets up a struggle with it because a "symptom" is by definition something "pathological"; something we should try to get rid of. In ACT, the aim is to transform our relationship with our difficult thoughts and feelings, so that we no longer perceive them as "symptoms." Instead, we learn to perceive them as harmless, even if uncomfortable, transient psychological events. Ironically, it is through this process that ACT actually achieves symptom reduction – but as a by-product and not the goal.
>
> *(p. 3)*

This point was critical in introducing ACT to Jane as a model for addressing her health anxiety, as one of her concerns was that people might think her physical symptoms were "all in her head." I worked to validate her experience of very real physical sensations, while simultaneously orienting her toward the ACT approach of mindfully experiencing her thoughts and feelings nonjudgmentally. In the case of health anxiety, sensations from the body are often interpreted as a "symptom" and initiate worry and rumination.

ACT for health anxiety: Program overview

To provide structure for our work together, I adapted the "Acceptance and Commitment Group Therapy (ACT-G) for Severe Health Anxiety" program developed by Eilenberg, Frostholm, and Kronstrand (2014). As originally designed, this program is quite comprehensive (ten sessions of three hours' duration) both in length and depth. Eilenberg et al. (2014) have produced an ACT-G manual to accompany the program, consisting of a short overview of each session, a detailed therapist guide for each session, participant handouts, and therapist instructions for the ACT exercises included in the program.

While originally developed for group settings led by two therapists, I modified the ACT-G material for 60–90 minute sessions with an individual athlete, while maintaining the predominantly experiential focus of ACT for health anxiety with many experiential exercises. The ten sessions are grouped into three phases: Creative Hopelessness, Willingness and Defusion, and Values and Committed Action. Sessions were conducted in person in my office at the USOPC Training Centre and remotely (via telephone and video consultation).

As described by Eilenberg et al. (2014), sessions 1–9 of the ACT-G program are delivered on a weekly basis, while session 10 is a booster session that may occur weeks after the ninth session. While Jane and I did progress through the ACT for health anxiety sessions in sequence, some sessions were combined (due to Jane's efficacy progressing through the program) such that the main components of the ACT-G program were adapted and delivered across seven sessions (60–90 minutes each). These sessions were interspersed with sport psychology consultations (60–90 minutes each) addressing performance readiness for training and competition. We typically worked together 2–3 times per month, over a period of six months, to complete the ACT for health anxiety program, with ongoing sessions as needed. As ACT is a foundational orientation influencing my sport psychology consultation, there was much overlap and complementarity across the health anxiety-focused sessions and more traditional sport psychology sessions. Jane appreciated that the ACT principles of mindfulness and values-guided action were relevant for both health anxiety and performance readiness, in that the skills she was learning could be flexibly applied to either context.

Session 1: Introduction

As described by Eilenberg et al. (2014), the purpose of the first session is to introduce the framework of ACT for health anxiety with a focus on initial motivation in relation to the work and willingness toward an experience-oriented approach. To facilitate understanding of health anxiety, I showed Jane the "increasing anxiety spiral" (Figure 8.1), which illustrates how thoughts, emotions and sensations interact and thereby maintain and enhance "normal" unpleasant sensations. In this model, sensations from the body are interpreted as a "symptom" and initiate worry and rumination. Attention is then influenced by the presence of illness

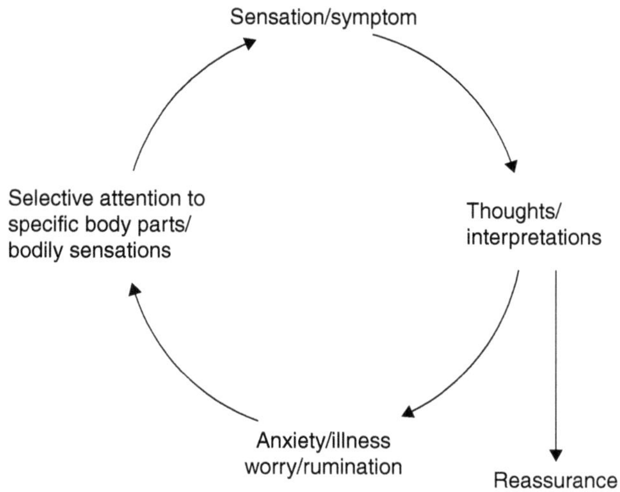

FIGURE 8.1 Increasing anxiety spiral (ACT for health anxiety)

worry and becomes increasingly focused on a specific body part. Increased awareness of specific physical sensations can increase the perception of them and therefore can easily lead to further concerns and confirm the assumption that the sensations are indeed "dangerous" (Eilenberg et al., 2014). Greater awareness of the "increasing anxiety spiral" can break this automatic cycle, leading to more effective interpretations and actions.

I informed Jane that a basic principal of ACT is that changes happen through experience and direct feeling in the moment. This meant that I would invite her to participate in exercises, some of which might be difficult and generate uncertainty and discomfort. I asked her to be as open as she could while engaging in the exercises, while remembering that she always had the option to opt out – even if the exercise was in progress.

We began with a mindfulness exercise ("Where do you want to go?") to further clarify Jane's reasons for engaging in our work together. In this exercise, I asked her to respond to questions such as "Why am I here?" and "Which direction do I want to move in?" (to begin addressing her values); "How do I respond to the idea of having to move?" and "What thoughts, feelings and body sensations arise?" (to address potential barriers); and "Am I willing to move in that direction with these barriers?" (to explore willingness and dedication).

As with all the ACT for health anxiety sessions, we concluded the first program session with a brief mindfulness exercise ("Where do you want to go?"). This exercise helped to set the stage for Jane's first homework assignment ("What do I really want my life to be about"), which I assigned at the end of the session. Eilenberg et al. (2014) note that this homework helps to clarify values, creating motivation and direction during the program.

Session 2: Introduction to ACT and mindfulness

The purpose of the second session is to provide an overall understanding of ACT and mindfulness, and to provide participants with some experience of both. I further introduced the essential concepts and clarified the focus and formal purpose of ACT and mindfulness practice (as applied to both health anxiety and performance readiness). Finally, I presented an overview of the entire ACT for health anxiety program.

We began this second session with a brief breathing space exercise, noting that this exercise would be repeated in connection with the presentation of mindfulness later in the session. I then followed up on Jane's homework assignment ("What do I really want my life to be about?") in terms of both content and process. Content questions included, "Are there new values or areas of your life of which you have become aware? Have you discovered that there may be a difference in how important a value is and how much you are acting on it?" Process questions included, "What are the barriers you've found in relation to having to do home assignments? What feelings, thoughts or sensations arose while doing the home assignments? How did you react to these?"

Jane identified several key values ("strong relationships" and "resilience") that would serve to guide her actions and decisions. Jane diligently completed her homework and didn't report any barriers to working on this assignment. She did note that examining her values revealed some experiential avoidance. While she is a rather social person, she realized that she occasionally passed up invitations to spend time with friends due to fatigue or to perceptions that her physical symptoms might flare up. She also noticed that preoccupation with health concerns affected her focus in training (e.g., "I hope I can complete today's workout").

As I couldn't improve on Eilenberg et al.'s (2014) eloquent description of the importance of values, I shared the authors' wording with Jane verbatim:

> While pursuing values we encounter pain, i.e. unpleasant thoughts, bodily sensations and emotions, such as illness worry. ACT assumes that pain is part of living a valuable and vital life but, through learning in our childhood and because of cultural norms, we have "learned" that we can avoid the pain through avoidance and control strategies. This works well in the short run, but in the long run, we often find that life is narrowed and that the pain may actually increase.
>
> *(p. 18)*

Next, I modified the ACT-G exercise "Take your mind for a walk" for use with Jane. This role-play activity was designed to emphasize the relationship Jane had with her thoughts. I invited Jane to imagine walking around while I played the role of her mind, in which I verbalized the thoughts and feelings Jane had shared with me about her health. Initially, I invited her to argue against me in the same way she might if she was having an internal dialogue with her thoughts about health anxiety. Next, I invited her to again take her mind for a walk, but this time, to leave her thoughts as a background commentary without arguing against them.

I extended this metaphor from the context of health anxiety to competition. Often, athletes hold the idea that they must have only positive thoughts, or that they're supposed to block out negative or unpleasant thoughts in order to perform well. I used the metaphor of taking her mind for a walk to introduce the concept that "there is a difference between thinking and attention" (Peter Haberl, personal communication, 2019). In a state of mindfulness, thoughts and feelings are observed as events in the mind, without over-identifying with them, and without reacting to them in an automatic, habitual pattern of reactivity. Mindfulness is not a practice in thought suppression; all thoughts or events are considered an object of observation. Once these thoughts or feelings are acknowledged, attention is directed back to the chosen target object (Bishop et al., 2004). Harris (2006) utilizes the difference between thinking and attention in his description of "defusion" (discussed later in this chapter) as the process of looking *at* thoughts, rather than *from* thoughts; noticing thoughts, rather than being caught up in thoughts, so that one can more flexibly aim attention at the present experience.

To further explain the difference between thinking and attention, an athlete might be asked to imagine a ball being thrown at her face. The athlete may have the thought, "I hope I don't get hit in the nose!" while simultaneously reaching out to catch the ball. The portion of the athlete's mind that leads her to reach for the ball is "attention," a concept that athletes easily grasp as distinct from the thoughts or feelings about the ball (Peter Haberl, personal communication, 2019). When training or competing, Jane didn't need to waste energy avoiding or getting tangled up in her thoughts. Rather, her job was to mindfully acknowledge the thoughts and feelings that might be distracting her from the present moment, then gently aim her attention at task-relevant cues. Instead of blocking out distracting thoughts, she could let them be there, as long as she aimed her attention in a way that helped her perform well. If the thoughts wanted to come along with her while training and competing, so be it. Her job was to aim her attention.

The concept of "aiming attention" (i.e., maintaining multisensory focus on immediate, current experience) is described by Bishop et al. (2004) in their definition of mindfulness from a Western psychological perspective. Bishop et al. (2004) define mindfulness as the self-regulation of attention, consisting of aiming attention, sustaining attention, regaining attention, and inhibiting elaborate processing. Similarly, as Dunne (2015) notes, the basic skills athletes may cultivate through formal training in Contemporary Mindfulness include: (1) holding an object in sustained, present-centered attention; (2) monitoring awareness for distractions (e.g., thoughts, feelings, sensations) in a non-judgmental fashion; (3) non-reactively disengaging from distractors; and (4) reorienting attention to the target object.

In addition to the attentional self-regulation aspects of mindfulness, Bishop et al. (2004) further define mindfulness as an intentional orientation to experience involving a commitment to maintaining an attitude of curiosity about where the mind wanders whenever it inevitably drifts away from the target object (e.g., experience distraction), as well as curiosity about the different objects within one's experience at any moment. All thoughts, feelings and sensations that arise are subject to observation. Thus, an athlete practicing mindfulness is not trying to produce a particular state, such as relaxation, or change what he or she is feeling in any way. Rather, the athlete is encouraged to just notice each thought, feeling, and sensation that arises in the stream of consciousness (Bishop et al., 2004). In this manner, a stance of acceptance is taken toward each moment of one's experience. Acceptance is defined as being experientially open to the reality of the present moment (Roemer & Orsillo, 2002). It involves a conscious decision to abandon one's agenda to have a different experience and an active process of "allowing" current thoughts, feelings, and sensations (Hayes, Strosahl, & Wilson, 2012). It is an active process in that the athlete chooses to take what is offered with an attitude of openness and receptivity to whatever occurs in the field of awareness (e.g., accept the distraction for what it is before reorienting attention). Thus, mindfulness can be conceptualized as a process of relating openly with experience. More simply, Kabat-Zinn (1990) defines mindfulness as the awareness that arises from paying attention, on purpose, in the present moment and non-judgmentally.

Jane was asked to continue practicing the breathing space exercise between sessions, both formally (as a sitting meditation) as well as during everyday activities, such as brushing teeth, during meals, and in between training repetitions as appropriate. Her homework assignment was to consider "What did I give up this week due to health anxiety?" The purpose of this exercise was to increase Jane's understanding of the costs of struggling with health anxiety. This also prepared her for the theme of the next session – creative hopelessness.

Session 3: How have you tried to manage your health anxiety?

The purpose of this session was to examine Jane's control strategies and experiences in coping with health anxiety. Jane and I collaboratively explored whether her previously used strategies had been effective in the short and long term in relation to living a values-based life.

We discussed Jane's experiences with practicing mindfulness and reviewed her homework. Jane described some of the things she had tried in order to solve or eliminate health anxiety. Typically, this would include ineffective strategies to either distract herself from unpleasant thoughts and feelings (doing homework, watching movies) or attempts to refute them ("I'm a tough athlete, I'm supposed to push through this"). Once we outlined her typical control strategies, we examined the most common triggers (unwanted feelings, sensations, etc.), how she characteristically responded to the unpleasant thoughts/feelings/sensations (such as illness worry), and the short-and long-term effects of these responses. The focus of this discussion was on the response rather than the trigger, with the goal of increasing Jane's understanding that it is avoidance that causes suffering, not the trigger of illness worry itself. Another way of stating this is that, while emotional pain is often quite unavoidable in human experience, suffering is optional (Pearson, Heffner, & Follette, 2010). Jane was suffering, and as do most humans, was engaging in some "experiential avoidance" to alleviate or avoid emotional pain. This experiential avoidance actually created additional suffering for Jane, as it further disrupted training and competition, and affected her relationships with friends and family.

Jane particularly liked the metaphor of control strategies as analogous to trying to dig herself out of a hole: The more she digs, the bigger the hole becomes. The problem is not the tool (the shovel) – it's the situation in which Jane was using it. She smiled in agreement when asked, "Are you ready to stop digging and do something else?"

Session 4: Control or values? Session 5: Willingness

I chose to combine sessions 4 and 5, as Jane easily grasped the concept of avoiding or controlling thoughts, feelings, and sensations (i.e., understanding that such attempts might lead her away from the life she wanted) and that it is preferable to meet thoughts and feelings with willingness.

Since Jane was still intermittently experiencing disruptive physical sensations during training (such as feeling atypically fatigued after intensive interval workouts), her sports medicine team conducted an EKG stress test to rule out heart abnormalities and tested her for potential underlying medical conditions such as Lyme disease. While testing suggested she had mononucleosis at some point, it was inconclusive as to when she'd contracted it. All other tests were negative. We examined her response to these physical sensations in the context of values-based living, rather than reacting with ineffective control strategies. As before, I validated her experience of these physical sensations, while inviting her to mindfully experience them nonjudgmentally.

Jane related a concern that these physical sensations might be in some way related to her parent's death when she was younger. Despite stating that she knew this was "probably irrational," this powerful thought contributed to her preoccupation with potential health abnormalities and was occasionally disruptive to her focus during training. This topic was explored across multiple sessions.

Jane and I reviewed the "Sports Bull's Eye" worksheet and dartboard (i.e., a sports version of the "Bull's Eye Values Survey"; Lundgren, Luoma, Dahl, Strosahl, & Melin, 2012; Larsen, Reinebo, & Lundgren, 2019) to further clarify what was meaningful to her both in sport and life. I emphasized that "willingness" doesn't mean she needed to like, want, enjoy, desire, or approve of something. Willingness means she'll allow it, make room for it, or let it be, in order to do something that she values (Harris, 2007).

We discussed in greater depth the concepts of pain versus suffering in terms of what Jane was willing to accept. The invitation to accept physical health difficulties does not refer to the suffering that comes from avoidance, but the natural pain or discomfort that is a part of life – in this case having a "noisy" body and worrying thoughts. Our bodies continually send signals that can be useful for survival. Much of this natural noise may be harmless, but if we give too much attention to it, we amplify it and may interpret it as dangerous symptoms.

I clarified that willingness does not mean passive acceptance of the situation or "giving up" – indeed, as an elite endurance athlete, Jane was used to (and even drew satisfaction from) a certain degree of pain as an intrinsic aspect of her sport. Jane's interpretation of her physical symptoms could lead to suffering, or she could be willing to accept the uncertainty and discomfort of her sensations.

Jane appreciated that this concept of willingness could be applied to both health anxiety and performance readiness. To practice greater willingness to experience painful sensations without intensifying them into suffering, we engaged in an ACT exercise utilizing acceptance and defusion strategies (Hayes, Strosahl, & Wilson, 2012) in which Jane was asked to hold an ice cube. Jane was reminded that this was a mindfulness technique, not a distraction or avoidance technique. As Jane held the ice in a clenched fist, bringing her attention to the sensations in her hand, she was asked to open up to these sensations, and to notice the difference between the sensations themselves and the story her mind was offering up about the sensations. Jane described two internal stories. Her mind alternated between the thoughts, "This is cold and painful; I want to drop the ice" and "I'm a tough athlete, I can take it, I won't put it down." Rather than reactively, automatically responding to the stories her mind was creating about the sensations, she learned to aim her attention on the sensations themselves. She was able to notice the sensations as just sensations (e.g., there was a centre to the sensations, and a periphery; the intensity of the sensations rose and fell in waves). Jane learned to make room for the sensations and reduce her struggle with them. She realized that the sensations couldn't overwhelm her or hurt her, and that she could stay present in the presence of unpleasant sensations. Jane began to apply this approach to both health anxiety and the pain she encountered in training and competition. Indeed, she reported that when she felt pain in a race, she was able to experience it mindfully, noticing the pain as bodily noise rather than responding ineffectively to the story her mind gave her about this sensation. She reported that this allowed her to more quickly and flexibly aim her attention at task-relevant cues. She also developed a more helpful, intentional story to interpret pain during a race (i.e., if she was in pain, then others must be in pain also). She stated, with evident satisfaction, that if competitors were going to beat her, they'd have to earn it – she'd make them suffer!

Session 6: Defusion. Session 7: You are more than your stories

As Jane was skilfully moving through the ACT for health anxiety program, I combined sessions 6 and 7. The purpose of session 6 is to introduce the concept of defusion. Intentionally creating distance from thoughts through defusion can help people to act on thoughts and feelings in line with their values – rather than use control and avoidance behaviors.

Cognitive fusion is one of the six core problems addressed in ACT. Harris (2007) notes that in cognitive fusion, people treat thoughts as reality, as truth; as important; as orders to be obeyed; and as wisdom (i.e., we assume 'thoughts' know best and we follow their advice).

Harris (2007) describes the strategy of defusion as looking *at* thoughts, rather than *from* thoughts; noticing thoughts, rather than being caught up in thoughts; and seeing thoughts as what they are, not as what they seem to be. He states that the aim of defusion is not to feel better, nor to get rid of unwanted thoughts; rather, the aim of defusion is to reduce influence of unhelpful cognitive processes upon behavior; to facilitate being psychologically present and engaged in experience; and to enhance psychological flexibility. Jane and I discussed defusion as a technique to approach thoughts and feelings more effectively. She then practiced a mindful thought observation exercise to begin distinguishing between having a thought and believing in a thought, and to see thoughts as thoughts and sensations as sensations (similar to the ice cube exercise previously described). She increasingly engaged in these exercises with willingness and intentionality, saying that they reinforced the concept of thinking vs. attention. She liked using the ACT skills to help manage her health anxiety as well as prepare for races. When she practiced mindfulness, she said that all she had to do was change the anchor of her attention (e.g., breathing during sitting meditation, sensations whenever they arose, or some task-relevant technical/tactical cue when training and competing) to fit the appropriate context.

I clarified for Jane that while the previous exercise was about achieving distance from her thoughts, the next exercise would be about her relationship with her thoughts about *herself*. This introduced the concept of "the observing self" (session 7). The observing self can detect and observe private experiences as nothing more than just experiences – to relate to a thought as just an idea and nothing else, thereby facilitating greater willingness to experience difficult feelings and observe thoughts without having to automatically react. By increasing contact with her observing self, Jane would become less invested in identifying herself with her thoughts, so that her whole identity would not have to depend on what 'her thoughts say about her'. As we engaged in various mindfulness exercises related to Jane's observing self, I drew her attention to the distinction between the thoughts that arise, and the self who observes those thoughts. From the perspective of this observing self, no thought is dangerous, threatening, or controlling (Harris, 2006). As Jane progressed through the ACT program, she reported responding more flexibly to bodily noise, with less automatic anxiety and fewer ineffective control strategies.

Session 8: What is valuable for you? Session 9: Living your values

Sessions 8 and 9 were combined to further clarify values and define specific value-based steps that could be taken going forward. "Value-based action" was introduced as an opportunity to expand Jane's repertoire with activities other than avoidance behavior, and control or excessive preoccupation with bodily sensations. We examined the key values that Jane identified in session 2 ("strong relationships" and "resilience"). Jane noted that examining her values revealed some experiential avoidance. As previously mentioned, Jane occasionally passed up invitations to spend time with friends due to fatigue. She also noticed that preoccupation with health concerns affected her focus in training. Through the program, when she became aware that health anxiety interfered with relationships, she began to act on her values by deciding not only to accept invitations to be with friends, but also being more intentionally present with them. When health sensations posed a challenge to training, she acted on her value of resilience to notice the story her mind created about these sensations and respond with greater psychological flexibility. Rather than trying to avoid or block out these sensations by "pushing through it," she instead reported acknowledging them with less judgment, then gently aiming her attention at task-relevant cues.

As an elite athlete, Jane was used to having sport-specific goals. I clarified the difference between goals and values, presenting values as a continuous choice, which are dynamic and take place in the present. This concept resonated with Jane. Endurance athletes typically have a "why" – a motivating reason to undergo arduous training and push themselves in competition. Jane's values connected with her motivation to be the best athlete she could be, which she subsequently demonstrated though consistent training and race performance.

During this phase of our work together, Jane reported that further medical evaluation revealed a diagnosis of Celiac disease, and that she was already feeling better by switching to a gluten-free diet. Over the next several months, she found that her troubling bodily sensations decreased, and she was able to train and compete with fewer restrictions. She did still occasionally experience fatigue, stomach pain, headaches, and sometimes heart palpitations, but when she became aware of these sensations, she reported doing better at mindfully observing them, without being as quick to judge or avoid them. She reminded herself of the values that she wanted to guide her actions, building on the work in sessions 8 and 9.

In line with session 10 (i.e., the 'booster' session; Eilenberg et al., 2014), we reviewed all of our work together and we also discussed potential future setbacks or obstacles. A common concern is that health anxiety sensations might return or worsen. I reminded Jane that the purpose of ACT is not necessarily symptom reduction but rather to enable her to live a vital and meaningful life, even when things are hard.

Reflections

During my work with Jane, I noticed moments when our interaction would lose vitality and when I would "lose my way." Inevitably, this was a result of my efforts to adhere too rigidly to the structure of the ACT for health anxiety program, rather than being more fully present with Jane. I also became aware of my tendency to fall into theoretical or intellectual discussions about issues, which served as a reminder to reconnect with the experiential nature of ACT. As I become more proficient in applying ACT, I will heed Harris' (2009) advice: "Be yourself; everyone else is already taken" (p. 3). Any missteps in my work with Jane were not due to the excellent program developed by Eilenberg et al. (2014); I simply needed to be more mindful about the here-and-now experience in our work together.

To mental performance and mental health consultants who wish to apply ACT in their own practice with athletes, I offer my colleague Peter Haberl's (2012) advice: "To think we can talk about mindfulness and then apply it when it matters most at the Games is probably wishful thinking. Mindfulness is a trainable skill, a skill that requires hard work, diligence, intentionality, and commitment" (p. 65). This is a useful axiom, as both practitioners and performers can benefit from daily mindfulness practice. The ACT program described in this case study serves as a valuable framework to work through different components associated with living a mindful, authentic, and satisfying life across different contexts, including elite sport.

Indeed, the case presented in this chapter reflects the service philosophy of the USOPC sport psychologists. As my colleague Sean McCann (2008) has stated, at the Olympic and Paralympic Games, everything is a performance issue. Since everything in the psychological life of the athlete can affect sustained competitive excellence and holistic well-being, we do not make an artificial distinction between clinical (counseling) services and educational/performance services. ACT, as applied in the preceding case, reflects this integrated approach. Jane learned skills allowing her to manage any re-emergence of health anxiety and facilitate consistent performance readiness.

I hope that this case illustrates the versatility of ACT and may benefit researchers, sport psychology practitioners, coaches, and students of sport psychology in supporting elite athlete mental health and performance.

References

Bishop, S., Lau, M., Shapiro, S., Carlson, L., Anderson, N., Carmody, J., ..., & Devins, G. (2004). Mindfulness: A proposed operational definition. *Clinical Psychology: Science and Practice 11*(3), 230–241.

Dunne, J. D. (2015). Buddhist styles of mindfulness: A heuristic approach. In B. D. Ostafin, M. D. Robinson, & B. P. Meier (Eds.), *Handbook of mindfulness and self-regulation* (pp. 251–270). New York, NY: Springer.

Eilenberg, T., Frostholm, L., & Kronstrand, L. (2014). *Acceptance and commitment group therapy (ACT-G) for severe health anxiety*. The Research Clinic for Functional Disorders and Psychosomatics, Aarhus University Hospital, Aarhus, Denmark.

Haberl, P. (2012). Dr. Peter Haberl, United States Olympic Committee. In M. Aoyagi & A. Poczwardowski (Eds.), *Expert approaches to sport psychology: Applied theories of performance excellence* (pp. 51–70). Morgantown, WV: Fitness Information Technology.

Harris, R. (2006). Embracing your demons: An overview of acceptance and commitment therapy. *Psychotherapy in Australia, 12* (4), 1–8.

Harris, R. (2007). Acceptance and Commitment Therapy (ACT) introductory workshop handout. Retrieved from www.actmindfully.com.au/

Harris, R. (2009). *ACT made simple*. Oakland, CA: New Harbinger.

Harris, R. (2011). *The confidence gap: A guide to overcoming fear and self-doubt*. Boston, MA: Trumpeter.

Harris, R. (2016). The single most powerful technique for extreme fusion. Retrieved from www.actmindfully.com.au/upimages/The_Single_Most_Powerful_Technique_for_Extreme_Fusion_-_Russ_Harris_-_October_2016.pdf

Hayes, S., Strosahl, K., & Wilson, K. (2012). *Acceptance and commitment therapy: The process and practice of mindful change*. New York, NY: Guilford.

Kabat-Zinn, J. (1990). *Full catastrophe living*. New York, NY: Random House.

Larsen, C. H., Reinebo, G., & Lundgren, T. (2019). Helping athletes clarify their values and become grounded in their sport venture (i.e. values and self as context). In K. Henriksen, J. Hansen, & C. H. Larsen (Eds.), *Mindfulness and acceptance in sport: How to help athletes perform and thrive under pressure*. New York, NY: Routledge.

Lundgren, T., Luoma, J., Dahl, J., Strosahl, K., & Melin, L. (2012). The bull's-eye values survey: A psychometric evaluation. *Cognitive and Behavioral Practice 19*(4), 518–526.

McCann, S. (2008). At the Olympics, everything is a performance issue. *International Journal of Sport and Exercise Psychology 6*, 267–276.

Nilsson, H., & Kazemi, A. (2016). From Buddhist sati to Western mindfulness practice: A contextual analysis. *Journal of Religion & Spirituality in Social Work: Social Thought 35,* 7–23. https://doi.org/10.1080/15426432.2015.1067582

Olendzki, A. (2013). The roots of mindfulness. In C. K. Germer, R. D., Siegel, & P. R. Fulton (Eds.), *Mindfulness and psychotherapy* (pp. 261–281). New York, NY: The Guilford Press.

Pearson, A., Heffner, M., & Follette, V. (2010) *Acceptance and commitment therapy for body image dissatisfaction.* Oakland, CA: New Harbinger.

Roemer, L., & Orsillo, S. M. (2002). Expanding our conceptualization of and treatment for generalized anxiety disorder: Integrating mindfulness/acceptance-based approaches with existing cognitive-behavioral models. *Clinical Psychology-Science & Practice 9,* 54–68.

United States Olympic and Paralympic Committee Mission Statement. Retrieved from www.teamusa.org/about-the-usopc

9

COACH'S INFLUENCE ON ATHLETES' MENTAL HEALTH IN TAIWAN

A case report

Frank J. H. Lu

Competitive sports contexts in Taiwan

Taiwan is a small island located in east-southern China of 35,808 square kilometers, which is inhabited by 23 million citizens of various ethnic groups: an original Chinese immigrant majority, an Aboriginal minority, and some new immigrants from Asia, Africa, Europe, Oceania, and America (Wikipedia, 2020). Although only a small island, Taiwan is ranked as the 21st economy body and the 15th GDP in the world. To develop and promote competitive sports in Taiwan, the Taiwanese government established a central sports regulatory authority named "Sports Council" (SC) in 1923. However, the early sports authority received little attention from the public and did not function well. After several times of reforms, the highest sports governing authority today is Sports Administration (SA) under the Ministry of Education (MOE, 2020).

For a long time, the competitive sport has been the most attractive form of sport in Taiwan. Especially, in the mid-twentieth century when a national youth baseball team won the Little League Baseball (LLB) championship in 1969 in the United States. The outstanding performance roused a nation's enthusiasm for competitive sports. For this reason, baseball became one of the most popular sports in Taiwan. Later, some Taiwanese players joined professional baseball teams in Japan, the US, Korea, and Taiwan which increased the popularity of baseball in Taiwan. In addition to baseball, basketball is also very popular due to a marked NBA influence. Many Taiwanese citizens watch the NBA from TVs and social media. They play basketball either for regular competition or recreational activities. In addition to baseball and basketball, Taiwanese also engage in many competitive sports such as archery, taekwondo, judo, track and field, weightlifting, volleyball, soccer, table-tennis, badminton, golf, swimming, shooting, and many others. There are many world-known sports stars in Taiwan such as Tai, Tzu-Ying (badminton), Yani Tseng (golf), Wei-Yin Chen and Wang, Chien-Ming (baseball), Chan, Yung-Jan and Su-Wei Hsieh (tennis), Kuo, Hsin-Chun (weight lifting), Chu Mu-Yen and Chen Shih-Hsin (taekwondo, 2004 Olympic Games gold medalists). The most regrettable thing for Taiwanese athletes to participate in international competition is that we are only allowed to use "Chinese Taipei" as an official name in the international sporting arena because of China's diplomatic policy.

As in many developed countries, engaging in competitive sport is potentially and financially rewarding in Taiwan. The reward system starts with governmental laws and regulations. For example, any Taiwanese athlete who wins a gold medal in the Olympic Games will earn 20 million Taiwanese dollars (equal to 666.000 US dollars or 645.000 Euro). Also, at every level of the school, the Sports Administration sets different regulations to reward coaches and athletes who perform outstandingly in the local, national, and international tournaments and competitions. Further, youth athletes earn monetary rewards from sports federations such as the Association of Tennis Professionals (ATP), Major League Baseball (MLB), Professional Golf Association (PGA), Ladies' PGA (LPGA), and many others. Moreover, Taiwanese athletes earn fame and reputation if they have outstanding athletic performance.

In Taiwan, the National Sports Training Center (NSTC) in Kaohsiung – a southern city of Taiwan, is the hub of elite sports. Established in 1976, the mission of the NSTC is to provide the best venues and programs for young athletes in Taiwan. The NSTC builds all sports facilities, dormitories, restaurants, and training programs for elite Taiwanese athletes to train regularly or intensively before any important competition such as world championships, Asian Games, and the Olympic Games. The coaches and athletes who train at NSTC will be not only offered free accommodation but also a temporary salary depending on their performance levels. Further, the NSTC recruits world best coaches from all over the world including Russia, China, Iran, Germany, Italy, Japan, Korea, and the US. The coaches' salary at NSTC is awarded according to their past coaching performance ranging from US 2000 to 10,000 dollars per month. The coaches are one of the core parts of elite sport. To be eligible as the national coaches at the NSTC, the local coaches must own a registered certificate from any sports federation. Further, he/she should demonstrate outstanding sports coaching performance every year as witnessed by his/her athletes having won important competitions or titles such as international tournaments or championships within the last year. There are more than 10,000 certified sports coaches in different sports in Taiwan. Thus, if anyone who wants to be a national coach at the NSTC, he/she needs to train his/her athletes at the local clubs/schools day and night, and even all year round. They have to sacrifice times with family and accompany athletes to compete either in local cities or abroad.

To establish a comprehensive environment for competitive sports in Taiwan, the NSTC also provides all types of sports science services for athletes. The NSTC has a Medical Center (MC) that offers health services for athletes including general medical care/treatment and athletic care/prevention. Also, NSTC hosts coaching education programs for coaches annually. Further, the NSTC establishes a Sport Counseling Center (SCC) which offers regular counseling services if athletes have any psychological disturbance. Also, the SCC regularly examine athletes' mental conditions when new members move to the NSTC. The SCC uses various psychological measures to evaluate athletes' psychological tendencies and mental health conditions. The measures range from sport-specific measures such as Sport Competition Anxiety Test (SCAT, Martens, 1977), Sport Confidence Inventory (SCI, Vealey, 1986), Athlete Burnout Questionnaire (ABQ, Raedeke & Smith, 2001) to general psychological measures such as State-Trait Anxiety Inventory (STAI, Spielberger, Gorssuch, Lushene, Vagg, & Jacobs, 1983), Beck Depression Inventory (Beck, Ward, Mendelson, Mock, & Erbaugh, 1961), and Profile of Mood State (POMS, McNair, Lorr, & Droppleman, & 1971).

Situating the author

Graduated from the University of North Carolina at Greensboro, USA, in 1998, I have been involved in sport psychology in Taiwan for many years. I work not only at the university with graduate students but also act as a consultant at the campuses, NSTC, and local sports clubs for athletes. While my research focuses on athletes' life stress, the psychology of sport injury, coaches' social support, and athletes' burnout, my applied experience involved helping both coaches and athletes with performance issues as well as mental health issues. In terms of mental health, I have helped athletes to use psychological measures such as ABQ, STAI, BDI to evaluate their mental states both on-campus and at the NSTC. As to coaches, the NSTC or sports associations in Taiwan invite me as a lecture/consultant to provide psychological services for them.

Case: A coach's leadership and how it influences athlete mental health

In the following, I will present the case of an archery coach at the NSTC. I visited NSTC several times and conducted an informal interview with him. Besides, I observed his training, collected data about his training histories, media reports, official documents, and public social media reports. Also, I informally interviewed some staff at the NSTC about the general information of my case. I took some photos and made field notes. I used a reflective interpretation method to analyze the data (Denzin & Lincoln, 2000). The following sections depict how a coach's leadership might influence athletes' mental health.

Mr. Wang: A national Olympic-level archery coach

Wang[1] is a 42-year-old male coach of the national archery team in Taiwan. When Wang was a middle school student, he was chosen by his PE teacher to practice archery for an extracurricular activity. After three months of training, he showed his talent and won a bronze medal in a local tournament. The first success inspired him to invest a great amount of time in archery training. Later, he entered a so-called "sports talent class" in the school, and continued archery training. After high school, he was admitted to enter a national sports university to continue his study and archery training. Through his high school to university, Wang did well in archery. He was chosen as a national delegate several times. However, when he came to the elite-level, it seemed very difficult for him to maintain a high rank in the Taiwanese archery arena. After he graduated from the university he was recruited at the athletic department by his alma mater university as an archery coach.

Wang is a mild and polite young man – qualities he has inherited from a traditional Chinese culture. Wang is responsible and diligent to coach his archery team. He coaches archery from early morning 6:30 to 08:00 and afternoon from 14:00 to 17:30 almost every day except Sunday. His patient and professional approach to training improved his athletes' performance and they won several times in the university-level tournaments and international competitions. Soon, he was recruited by Taiwan Archery Association (official name is "Chinese Taipei Archery Association") who assigned him as a head coach for the national archery team from 2003 to 2020. He led the Taiwanese national archery team to participate in numerous Asian Games, International Archery Championships, Asian Archery Championships, and the Olympic Games.

Before the Olympics

In the years 2014–2016, Wang was recruited as a national archery coach. This time he coached three male and three female archers to participate in the 2016 Brazil summer Olympic Games. To prepare this XXXI Olympiad in Rio De Janerio, the Taiwanese Archery Association recruited the best archers from every corner of Taiwan. Wang and his team members, including six archers and two assistant coaches, entered the NSTC six months before the 2016 Olympic Games. They set six-months training schedules and competition plans. The preparation for the 2016 Olympic Games was a long-lasting work for Wang and the team members. Although some of the archers had experiences in international competitions, most of them would compete in the Olympic Games for the first time. Adding to the team members' psychological burdens, the government and the citizens had very high expectations for their performance in the upcoming Olympic Games because the Taiwanese national archery team had excellent records in the previous Olympiad. Newspapers and social media reported their training and frequently asked coaches and athletes about their goals and expectations for the upcoming Olympic Games. To reduce pressure on the athletes, Wang blocked all the reporters' interviews before the Olympic Games. Also, to comfort team members' minds, he communicated with team members that the preparation process is the most important thing for them to focus on. His philosophy about winning and losing is "do your best, and let God decide the final results."

By this "step by step" manner, the Taiwanese archery team experienced peaceful training before the 2016 Olympic Games. However, even in the most ordinary training life, problems may occur, and so they did. The first example was that of a male archer who crashed seriously in a motorcycle accident two months before the Olympic Games. The unexpected traffic accident hurt his right shoulder, bruised some parts of the body, and two palms. For this accident, Mr. Wang banned the athletes from using a motorcycle as a transportation tool even for short distances. He took this injured archer to visit the doctor for a good treatment, and carefully supervised the recovery speed to provide appropriate training.

The other accident example was that of a female archer who comes from a single-parent family. Her parents divorced two years ago. She lived with her mother and away from her gamble-loving and drunk father. Her father harassed her mother quite often during the Olympic training period. Although a family matter and not directly related to sport, her father's behavior disturbed the athlete. When she talked to her mother on the phone, the athlete was sad and unfocused. Mr. Wang was aware of her mood disturbance and understood her situation. He comforted her and referred her to sport psychology counseling at SCC of the NTSC. At the same time, he used his social relationship to visit her father and tried to persuade him through a "patriotic" pep-talk to help his daughter during the Olympic preparation. To persuade the father, Mr. Wang described how he could be proud of his daughter's delegation for the Olympic Games. Mr. Wang also asked some friends to help the father to solve his troubles. The drunk and gamble-loving man finally accepted his suggestions after many visits, and went back a 'normal life', not only by avoiding to harass his wife but also by taking work at the local factory and keeping a low profile. Soon, the female archer became mood steady and continued her training.

In addition to these two unexpected troubles, there were also some minor disturbances in the team. Some members experienced staleness because of long and tedious training. In this case, Mr. Wang allowed some team members to adjust their training schedules if they didn't feel well. Absence in training at the NSTC is a serious violation which may cause disqualification for the national teams. However, this was not the case for the archery team because they had a considerate head coach. Mr. Wang understood that long-term training might cause athletes' tiredness and staleness. To minimize this, he occasionally allowed for time off and he set goals for everyday training. Also, before every training, he explained the objectives and the processes of the training. If any archer questioned the plan, he patiently explained or adjusted according to each archer's need. Therefore, his training is flexible, goal-directed, and characterized by reciprocal communication.

During the Olympics

During the 2016 Olympic Games, it was a very challenging battle. All international competitors improved quite a lot. So it was not so easy to win at any single match. The Taiwanese male archers did not perform as well as previous records, neither in men' single nor in group competitions. However, the female won a bronze medal in the group competition. Although performance did not quite reach expectations, the 2016 Taiwanese archery team experienced harmony in training and competition. Under Mr. Wang's leadership, the team members accomplished the mission that they were given by the nation. No interpersonal conflicts, depressions, or frustrations occurred in the 2016 Olympic Games. All team members remembered that they had worked together, shared joyful moments, and mutual supports.

After the Olympics

After the 2016 Olympic Games, all archery team members went back to their original schools and institutions. They met sometimes for a birthday party or occasional social gathering. All archery athletes continued to train at their respective schools or institutions because they are still young. They expect to come back for the next Olympiad.

Reflections

The Taiwanese archery coach's case brings lots of implications for the mental health in elite sport. The most salient part is that coach's leadership might influence athletes' mental health, even in a top-level competition such as the Olympic Games. In facing the highly competitive arena, most athletes experience pressures from personal, social, contextual, and interpersonal interactions. Some athletes experience conflicts because of team members' competition or feel lonely, and boring because of monotonous training, or frustration because of coaches' rigid, tight, and inflexible training schedule. These experiences are unhealthy for elite sport. According to World Health Organization (WHO), mental health is defined as "a state of well-being in which every individual realizes his or her own potential, can cope with the normal stresses of life, can work productively and fruitfully, and is able to contribute to her or his community" (Galdersi, Heinz, Kastru, Beezhold, & Sartorius, 2015).

In the present case, Mr. Wang did a good job in the 2016 Olympic Games to protect his team members from excessive training pressure, maintaining a steady mood to prepare for the Olympic Games, and cope with any stress from personal, contextual, or social sources. His leadership enabled his team members to perform well in the 2016 Olympic Games.

Coaches' multiple roles and responsibilities

Mr. Wang's role and responsibilities in elite sport are multiple. I find the Chelladurai (2007) multidimensional model of sport leadership is meaningful as a basic framework (see Figure 9.1) to explain his leadership. He uses his professional knowledge to provide quality practice for his archers (autocratic). But he will communicate to his team members about why they should train as scheduled (instruction and training). Besides, if any archer is tired of training he will try to understand the reasons behind tiredness and provided alternative activities (social support/democratic). He set goals for his team members to motivate them to engage in necessarily harsh physical training (feedback). No matter whether his team members are inexperienced or experienced athletes, he teaches them psychological skills training (PST) before and during training or competition. To increase coaching efficiency, he regularly participates in job-training, so he learns updated knowledge for training. Also, based on his careful observations, he takes action to solve team members' problems such as recovery after a motorcycle accident or a family conflict (social support). Thus, Mr. Wang's leadership seems to deeply influence the team members' mental health during the 2016 Olympic Games.

Based on Mr. Wang's educational and sporting background, we can see his leadership is influenced by many factors. First, his earlier archery background and education experience make him a knowledgeable and mature coach in archery. Also, his personality, mostly influenced by culture and Chinese tradition, makes him a considerate and caring coach. The cultural influences also include the Taiwanese government's sports policy, NSTC, citizen's passion for sports, sports tradition, reward system, and societal atmosphere.

Chelladurai's (2007) multidimensional model of sport leadership proposed cohesion, performance, and satisfaction as the major outcomes of the sport leadership. However, in my model, I proposed mental health is one of the potential outcomes of sport leadership. As it is illustrated, the culture influences the archery coach's personality, education systems, and sports environments that allow him to be a national coach at the NSTC and his positive leadership. His positive leadership influences his training arrangements and interactions with athletes, and his supportive behavior during Olympic preparation and competition. Consequently, positive leadership not only led to athletes' positive mental health but also performance and

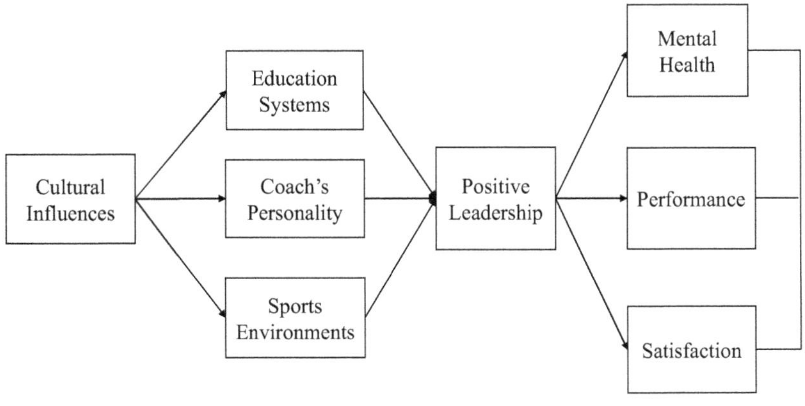

FIGURE 9.1 Schematic presentation of the mental health in elite sport in Taiwan

satisfaction. My model thus extends Chelladurai's (2007) concept and suggests that positive leadership is key to athletes' mental health. I hope future studies might examine how coaches' leadership influences athletes' mental health.

Practical applications

My case reports how a Taiwanese archery coach's leadership influenced athletes' mental health in elite sport. However, this case did not apply detailany specific intervention, nor did it evaluate what program would be effective to change an athlete's mental health from a poor to a positive condition. My case, in contrast, reports that coaches' leadership is important in enhancing or promoting athletes' mental health, especially, in a highly competitive setting. Sport psychologists or practitioners might apply my case to their coaching efficacy program. They can use my case as a backdrop to analyze which coaching behaviors are the most beneficial to protect athletes' mental health in their specific contexts, and how to cultivate coaches' positive leadership.

Conclusion

Mental health in elite sports is a prominent issue. To echo current professional appeals from the International Society of Sport Psychology (Henriksen et al., 2019; Schinke et al., 2017), I use a Taiwanese archery coach at the NSTC in Taiwan as an example to describe how a coach's leadership influences athletes' mental health.

Note

1 Wang is a pseudonym to protect the case's privacy. Also, the age and sport has been changed to secure a level of anonymity. The story combines several persons' encounters at the NSTC.

References

Beck, A. T., Ward, C. H., Mendelson, M., Mock, J., & Erbaugh, J. (1961) An inventory for measuring depression. *Archives of General Psychiatry 4*, 561–571.

Chang, K. H, Lu, F. J. H., Chyi, T., Hsu, Y. W., Chan, S. W., & Wang, E. T. W. (2018). Examining the stress-burnout relationship: The mediating role of negative thoughts. *Peer J. 5*(1), e4181. DOI 10.7717/peerj.4181.

Chelladurai, P. (2007). Leadership in sports. In G. Tennenbaum & R. C. Eklund (Eds.), *Handbook of sport psychology* (3rd., pp. 113–135). Hoboken, NJ: Wiley.

Chiu, S. S., Hsu, Y. W., Chiu, Y. H., Chou, C. C., Gill, D. L., & Lu, F. J. H. (2020). Seeking positive strengths in buffering athletes' life stress-burnout relationship: The moderating roles of athletic mental energy. *Frontiers in Psychology 10*, 1–12. doi: 10.3389/fpsyg.2019.03007.

Chyi, T., Lu, F. J. H., Wang, E. T. W., Hsu, Y. W., & Chang, K. H. (2017). Prediction of life stress on athletes' burnout: The dual role of perceived stress. *Peer J. 15*(6), e4213. DOI 10.7717/peerj.4213.

Denzin, N. K., & Lincoln, Y. S. (2000). *Handbook of qualitative research*. London: Sage Publications Inc.

Galdersi, S., Heinz, A., Kastru, M., Beezhold, J., & Sartorius, M. (2015). Toward a new definition of mental health, *World Psychiatry 14*(2): 231–233. DOI: 10.1002%2Fwps.20231.

Henriksen, K., Schinke, R., Moesch, K., McCann, S., Parham, W. D., Larsen, C. H., & Terry, P. (2019). Consensus statement on improving the mental health of high performance athletes. *International Journal of Sport and Exercise Psychology 18*(5), 553–560.

Lu, F. J. H., & Hsu, E.Y. W. (2013). Injured athletes' rehabilitation beliefs and subjective well-being: The contribution of hope and social support. *Journal of Athletic Training 48*(1), 92–98. DOI: 10.4085/1062-6050-48.1.03.

Lu, F. J. H., Hsu, Y. W., Chan, Y. S., Cheen, J. R., & Kao, K. T. (2012). Assessing college student-athletes' life stress: Initial measurement development and validation. *Measurement in Physical Education and Exercise Science 16*(4), 254–267. DOI:10.1080/1091367X.2012.693371.

Lu, F. J. H., Lee, W. P., Chang, Y. K., Chou, C. C., Hsu, Y. W., Lin, J. H., & Gill, D. L. (2016). Interaction of athletes' resilience and coaches' social support on the stress-burnout relationship: A conjunctive moderation perspective, *Psychology of Sport and Exercise 22*, 202–209.

Lu, F., Gill, L., Yang, M., Lee, P., Hsu, Y., Chiu, Y., & Kuan, G. (2018). Measuring Athletic Mental Energy (AME): Instrument development and validation. *Frontiers in Psychology 9*, 2363. DOI:10.3389/fpsyg.2018.02363.

Martens, R. (1977). Sport Competition Anxiety Test. IL: Human Kinetics Publishers.

McNair, D. M., Lorr, M., & Droppleman, L. F. (1971). *Manual for the profile of mood states*. San Diego, CA: Educational and Industrial Testing Services.

Meehan, H. L., Bull, S. J., Wood, D. M., & James, D. V. B. (2004). The overtraining syndrome: A multi-contextual assessment. *The Sport Psychologist, 18*, 154–171.

MOE (2020). *Sports Administration, Ministry of Education*, retrieved from www.sa.gov.tw/English/index?n=50 on May 2, 2020.

Raedeke, T. D., & Smith, A. L. (2001). Development and preliminary validation of an athlete burnout measure. *Journal of Sport & Exercise Psychology 23*, 281–306. doi: 10.1123/jsep.23.4.281.

Schinke, R. J., Stambulova, N. B., Si, G., & Moore, Z. (2017). International society of sport psychology position stand: Athletes' mental health, performance, and development. *International Journal of Sport and Exercise Psychology 16*(6), 622–639. DOI: 10.1080/1612197X.2017.1295557.

Spielberger, C. D., Gorsuch, R. L., Lushene, R., Vagg, P. R., & Jacobs, G. A. (1983). *Manual for the State-Trait Anxiety Inventory*. Palo Alto, CA: Consulting Psychologists Press.

Vealey, R. S. (1986). Conceptualization of sport-confidence and competitive orientation: Preliminary investigation and instrument development. *Journal of Sport Psychology 8*, 221–246. DOI: https://doi.org/10.1123/jsp.8.3.221

Wikipedia (2020). *Taiwan*, retrieved from https://en.wikipedia.org/wiki/Taiwan on 2 May 2020.

10

COLLABORATIVE CASE MANAGEMENT

Supporting mental health in the UK's high performance sport system

Samuel Cumming, Sarah Cecil, and Amanda Gatherer

Acknowledgements

The authors would like to acknowledge the English Institute of Sport's Mental Health Expert Panel (Professor Alan Currie, Dr Amanda Gatherer, and Dr Allan Johnston), Dr Craig Ranson and Dr Rod Jaques for their work as members of the Mental Health Team. We would also like to thank the practitioners who worked with the Mental Health Expert Panel on the cases which inspired this chapter and have not been mentioned by name to maintain the anonymity of these cases.

Introduction

The following case study is presented to illustrate some of the mental health support available to athletes within the High Performance System (HPS) in the UK. It also demonstrates a recommended approach to supporting an athlete in crisis whilst outside the UK. Whilst this case study draws on some themes from real cases from the HPS, Amy (the athlete described here) and the details of her case are fictional. They are presented to illustrate some of the key challenges faced by practitioners in the high performance system and reflect some important lessons. This chapter has been reviewed by key individuals from a number of sports involved in some of the cases which formed the inspiration for this chapter, to ensure that the anonymity of any related cases is maintained. Such use of fictional case studies to illustrate a process, intervention or approach is not a novel concept (Bathgate et al., 2013; Iles & Cranfield, 2004).

The context

Before describing the case itself it is worth outlining some background and context about the UK and the approach to providing mental health support via the EIS. Following the 2016 Olympic and Paralympic Games in Rio de Janeiro a Culture Health Check (CHC) was carried out by UK Sport to understand the cultural landscape of each National Governing Body (NGB) supported by UK Sport funding (UK Sport, 2018). The results of the CHC, alongside an independent Duty of Care in Sport Review by Baroness Tanni Grey-Thompson (2017) and a number of high-profile athletes sharing their struggles with mental health demonstrated a need for a more concerted and concentrated focus in this area. Concurrently, a similar increase in activity to support the mental health of elite athletes has been seen across the world of elite sport, particularly in Australia (Portch, 2019), the United States (NCAA, 2017) and in international bodies like the International Olympic Committee (Reardon et al., 2019).

The response from UK Sport to the results from the CHCs across sports was to develop a Mental Health Steering Group (MHSG) which developed a bespoke Mental Health Strategy. A major part of this strategy was to establish a centralised EIS Mental Health Team (MHT). The purpose of the MHSG & EIS MHT is to promote a sustainable High Performance System where all people have the best opportunity to have Positive Mental Health and ensure there is appropriate support for those experiencing mental health problems. A key group within the EIS MHT was the EIS Mental Health Expert Panel (MHEP) – a group of expert mental health professionals (clinical psychologists and sport psychiatrists) with significant experience of working in elite sport available to offer advice and guidance to the HPS on matters relating to mental health. The Panel were recently formed at the time of the case study described in this chapter. See Figure 10.1 for a visual representation of these groups.

The Mental Health Strategy devised by the MHSG defines both mental health problems and positive mental health in accordance with the World Health Organisation, as defined in Chapter 1.

It is also worth noting that, in the United Kingdom (UK), the title of 'Sport and Exercise Psychologist' is protected by the Health and Care Professions Council (HCPC) and registered status can be obtained by two routes; through the British Psychological Society (initial training as a psychologist, who specialises in sport) or through the British Association of Sport and Exercise Sciences (initial training as a sport scientist, who specialises in psychology). At present the EIS employs practitioners who have attained or are working towards HCPC registration via either route.

Case

Amy was a 24-year-old female athlete and an established member of the senior squad of her sport, on track to represent Great Britain at the Olympic Games in Tokyo. She had been competing in the sport since the age of 14, competed for Great Britain as a Junior athlete and achieved international success throughout her time in this sport's age-group categories. The sport described her as a potential medal-winning prospect in Tokyo. She lived alone with a very limited support network having relocated to train full-time with her sport which was a significant distance from home. Being part of the programme required Amy to spend periods of the year outside the UK at training camps and competitions. Amy had a history of moderate depression and anxiety with some panic attacks, first experienced during a stressful exam period at school and initially managed through sessions of cognitive behavioural therapy (CBT). She flagged this history with her NGB doctor and sport psychologist during her induction onto the senior programme three years ago; at that stage she described her mental

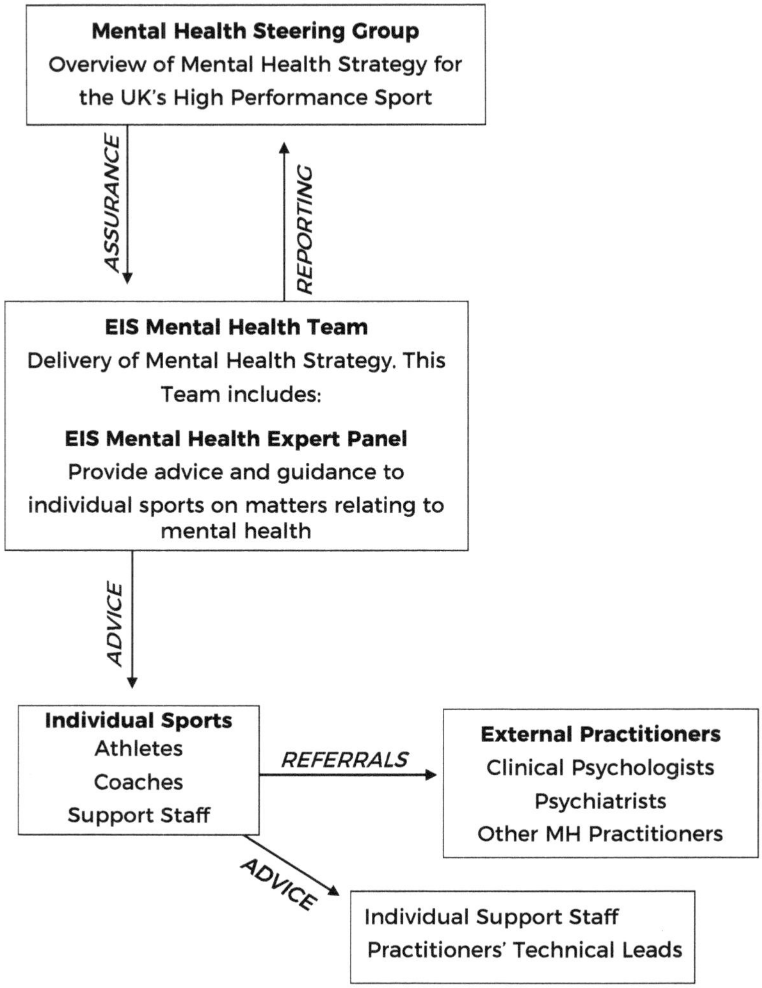

FIGURE 10.1 Visual representation of the various groups set up to support mental health in the UK High Performance Sport System

health problems as well-managed and had not experienced any elevated symptoms whilst training and performing in her chosen sport.

Amy continued to train and compete for Great Britain in her sport for three years after her initial induction, which brings this case almost to the present day. Shortly before departing for a training camp with her sport a close friend from outside Amy's sport died unexpectedly. This triggered an overwhelming sense of anxiety and a lack of control for Amy. The last time she had experienced these feelings at this intensity was shortly before experiencing a panic attack. This response was not known to the coaches or support staff within her sport, or anyone else outside of sport. She did not disclose her feelings of increased anxiety or lack of control prior to leaving for the training camp; instead sharing with her coaches and support staff that she was looking forward to an opportunity to 'escape home' of a few weeks and focus on her training.

The event and immediate response

Half-way through the camp Amy recognised the feelings of being overwhelmed, anxious and struggling to maintain control and she had a panic attack in the bathroom. When her roommate noticed that something was wrong and went to go and check on her, Amy asked her to get hold of the sport psychologist or the physiotherapist, with whom she had a good relationship. Amy's roommate was able to call both practitioners whilst she sat with Amy in the bathroom.

The immediate response from the psychologist and physiotherapist was to contain Amy, praise her for having sought their support, see if any immediate medical support was required following the panic attack and to check on the well-being of her roommate. The psychologist asked Amy about her current anxiety levels, how she had experienced the panic attack and what she had found helpful from her previous CBT sessions in managing them. The psychologist also advised Amy that, because of concerns for her safety, the psychologist would need to make a few other people aware to seek some additional support. There was no team doctor on this training camp but Amy agreed to the physiotherapist providing an update to the team doctor so that she could assess that Amy was safe and to start to arrange a referral on Amy's return to the UK, whilst Amy continued to talk with the psychologist. At the EIS all practitioners (e.g., physiotherapists, strength and conditioning coaches, psychologists, etc.) have a Technical Lead (TL) who is available to provide support and guidance. The TLs for psychologists also provide supervision. The psychologist also agreed with Amy that she would speak with her TL to agree some appropriate next steps. In the meantime, when they were confident in Amy's safety for the next few hours, the psychologist and physiotherapist agreed to check in with her the next morning and encouraged her to continue to speak with them. The psychologist had recently attended a targeted Mental Health First Aider education session for EIS staff, which she reported as helping guide her response in the moment.

Immediately after speaking with Amy the psychologist and physiotherapist debriefed the situation and agreed that they were both comfortable with their response and Amy's safety and her roommate's well-being. The psychologist then called her TL for advice, guidance and to seek any additional suggestions for next steps. The psychologist's TL agreed that her response had been appropriate and recommended speaking with a member of the EIS MHEP to fully debrief the practitioners' immediate response and agree appropriate next steps. After contacting the EIS's lead for mental health a call was arranged that evening with a member of the EIS MHEP.

The Panel member discussed the initial response and advised on an immediate support plan. This consisted of regular check-ins for Amy with the psychologist and physiotherapist during the camp, space to discuss the work from her former CBT sessions, a plan for assessment and psychological support on return to the UK. The Panel member also advised the psychologist to ensure that, as they were outside the UK and given the potential risk of another panic attack, the emergency response procedure in the country was known. It was also important to agree how the support team at the camp would respond in the event of an emergency, and also to discuss options for Amy to return to the UK early if required and safe to do so. Finally, the Panel member agreed to identify a suitable mental health practitioner to carry out an assessment of Amy when she returned to the UK in order to inform ongoing support. In the UK Sport HPS all high performance athletes in receipt of an Athlete Performance Award are supported with medical insurance cover (which provides parity for physical and mental health cover). This process is initiated by a doctor's referral.

At their scheduled check-in the next morning Amy told the psychologist that she felt unable to continue on the camp. She gave her consent for the psychologist to discuss the situation with the Performance Director so that return travel to the UK could be arranged. With the Performance Director they agreed that the psychologist would travel to the airport with Amy later that day, ensuring she got on her flight safely. They had also arranged for a UK-based member of the support staff to meet her at the airport in the UK and accompany her to their EIS site to see the NGB doctor and initiate the referral process. With Amy's consent the doctor liaised with the same EIS MHEP member who had spoken with the sport psychologist and recommended a suitable, local clinical psychologist for an initial assessment. Following this assessment the local clinical psychologist recommended Amy start a six week course of regular CBT with two follow-up sessions in the next six months. These sessions would focus on identifying, challenging, and changing unhelpful thoughts, feelings and behaviours which led to Amy's panic attacks, especially those relating to anxiety and a lack of control.

Whilst discussing plans to return to the UK with the Performance Director and psychologist Amy was asked how she would like the rest of the team to be informed about her leaving the camp. Amy said that she was happy for the rest of the team to be told that she had left the camp following concerns about her mental health and to seek support back in the UK. The Performance Director shared this with the rest of the group at a team meeting later that day.

Actions after the event

The Performance Director described the event as a prompt for the sport to be more aware about mental health, both the area in general and specifically relating to the mental health of their athletes. The response at the camp had been very positive; the psychologist and physiotherapist had reacted calmly and provided excellent support, maintaining the safety of the athlete as the main priority. Contacting the EIS MHEP provided assurance that the best steps had been taken and the response to returning the athlete home had been quick and well-organised. The Performance Director's concern was that the situation may have been different if Amy had disclosed this to other members of staff who have had less training in triaging and referring mental health problems. This led to a follow-up call with the EIS Mental Health lead to identify what additional support was available.

At this time the EIS MHT had developed a mental health awareness workshop which was being delivered across the High Performance System. This workshop focussed on allowing participants to feel more comfortable and confident in talking about mental health. It covered general mental health awareness (including definitions, ways to talk about mental health, potential signs that someone may be struggling), how to promote positive mental health (including the importance of self-care) and responding to real life concerns (including sport-specific and general referral pathways and some scenario discussions). These sessions were typically delivered collaboratively with a member of the sport's support staff which enables the session to be made more bespoke for the audience. It was agreed that, as part of the support provided by the EIS in this case, an adapted version of this awareness workshop would be delivered in the sport. This workshop was delivered by a member of the EIS MHT and the sport's psychologist and was designed to spend longer focussing on the 'responding to real life concerns' section. This workshop also provided an opportunity for the sport psychologist to outline the sport's referral procedure and who to talk to if anyone had concerns about their own or someone else's mental health.

The EIS Mental Health Lead also recommended a group debrief and decompression of the event, facilitated by a clinical psychologist. The Performance Director reported that a number of athletes and staff had been significantly impacted after witnessing Amy's panic attack and Amy's subsequent disclosure of what she had experienced; a mixture of concern for Amy and distress that they had 'missed something'. Shortly after Amy's departure from the training camp the sport's support staff had noticed that Amy's roommate from the training camp had been particularly affected. The decompression session brought together those involved in the immediate response along with those impacted subsequently (including her coach and on-camp roommate) to make sense of the event and discuss the impact on them in a safe space. A clinical psychologist was chosen to facilitate the session in order to provide a level of expertise in normalising the group's response to witnessing or hearing about a panic attack, their own response in the moment and to discuss what may trigger memories of the experience. This debrief also took place with Amy's consent.

Finally, roughly a month after Amy's return to the UK, the EIS MHT arranged for the clinical psychologist who carried out Amy's initial assessment and subsequent treatment to lead a team formulation to help those working closely with the athlete to understand her experience and needs. Specifically the group was formed of the psychologist and physiotherapist who provided the first response, the doctor, Performance Director and Amy's coach. This formulation followed the '5 Ps' approach (see Figure 10.2 for an illustrative example with minimal detail), based on the British Psychological Society's (2015) recommendations and a document developed by the Northumberland, Tyne and Wear NHS Foundation Trust (2018).

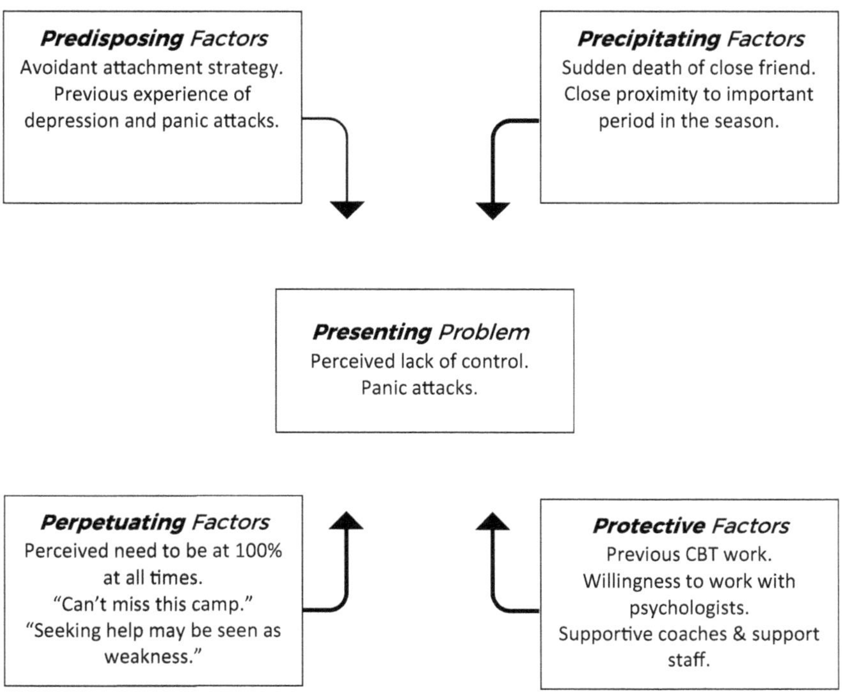

FIGURE 10.2 Illustrative example of a completed '5 P' formulation

The aim of the formulation session was to understand Amy from a variety of perspectives and also to ensure a shared understanding for those involved of the support Amy needed (Bickley, Rogers, Bell, & Thoms, 2016). The formulation was also carried out with Amy's consent with the intention of supporting her transition back into full-time training in an appropriately supportive and understanding environment. It also led to agreement of a safe-travel plan for all future trips.

Reflections

Coming at a relatively early stage in the development of the EIS MHT and MHEP this case provided a number of lessons which have informed their ongoing approach to supporting the mental health of those in the HPS. These lessons relate to the role of the EIS MHEP, the importance of proactive planning, content for ongoing education and recommendations made to sports when planning their mental health strategies.

First, this case highlighted the importance of sports having in place a clearly defined and well communicated referral process. This allows athletes and staff to feel more confident that, in the event of a mental health crisis, anyone from the sport would know who to speak to. In addition, when travelling abroad it is important for athletes and staff to know any changes to the referral process (if different to the 'at home' process). Ideally sports would also have a 'fitness to travel' protocol which incorporates consideration of mental health. The EIS MHEP are available to support sports in the development of these protocols, which may include developing a formal process to determine if someone is safe to travel. The EIS MHT include a section on the particular sport's referral process in all mental health awareness sessions.

Similarly, a clear understanding of who the EIS MHEP is and how to access them was a significant lesson from this case. The in situ response by the sport psychologist was good (her priority was the athlete's well-being at all times, she discussed what the athlete recalled from her previous CBT interventions, and maintained clear communication of next steps and the bounds of confidentiality) and her debrief with the Panel member did not make her change any of her actions. However, the value of having someone with experience to talk to and provide guidance cannot be underestimated. This was achieved both through the psychologist contacting her Technical Lead and by gaining access to the EIS MHEP. This has emphasised the importance of raising awareness across the HPS of the existence of the EIS MHEP and the kind of support they could offer in similar cases.

Next, the value of proactive steps to promote mental health awareness was evidenced by this case. Education sessions can help with this. These sessions can help to 'myth bust' some concerns about mental health. Although not relevant in this case, the idea that asking someone about self-harm or suicide will increase the risk of that person attempting it is a misconception (Enyan et al., 2014; Gould et al., 2005), is often met by surprise when it is presented in these education sessions. It is important that, in cases where this concern is relevant, people feel sufficiently confident to ask the appropriate questions in the appropriate way to determine risk. Also, it is anticipated that if a system can become more aware about mental health, understand the concept in a consistent way, share the same language when speaking about it, it is more able to promote an environment where people feel more open to sharing their experiences and seeking help when needed. Again, in this case it was helpful that Amy had built up sufficiently strong relationships with the psychologist and physiotherapist ask for their support.

The use of team formulation was another lesson from this case. Running a team formulation with key support personnel (with the athlete's consent and led by the mental health practitioner that they have been working with) is a significant advance in the support provided to the individual athlete and others in the sport. The team formulation combines the work carried out between the athlete and their therapist (including the psychological paradigm and underlying theory) with the 'real life' observations and experiences of those who work most closely with the athlete (Bickley et al., 2016). This keeps all key individuals on 'the same page', with a shared understanding of the athlete's needs and experiences and can support their reintegration back into the sport. It also helps the sport to recognise what changes may be necessary to make to ensure that the athlete is appropriately supported as they return to full-time training. This may include a better understanding of the athlete's boundaries, triggers to look out for, language to use, appropriate behaviours of coaches and support staff and specific behaviours to look out for from the athlete.

The impact of the athlete's disclosure on those around her provided another lesson from this case. The emotional reaction from other athletes, coaches, and support staff who had been informed about the case was significant. The concern and distress experienced by these individuals were described above. It is easy to assume that all attention should focus on the individual who has made the disclosure or been in crisis, however this case provided a reminder of the ripple effect of concern for those around the individual. The sport supported these individuals by arranging a facilitated 'decompression and debrief' session led by a clinical psychologist to discuss the impact (separate from the team formulation described in the previous paragraph). This role modelling of sharing experiences and feelings is a good indicator of the open and supportive culture within this particular sport.

Finally, this case demonstrates the importance of consent. In matters relating to disclosures about self-harm or suicidal ideation the concept of consent can be a cause for anxiety. There is often concern that if an individual shares information that suggests they are at risk to themselves or others they would not want anyone else to know. This leads to the individual receiving the disclosure carrying it on their own. However, it is important to understand confidentiality cannot be maintained if there is risk of harm to the individual or someone else, in order to seek the appropriate support. Some people explicitly ask for the information not to be shared any further. In this case the athlete was receptive to the psychologist explaining that, in order to provide the best support, she needed to share this information. Indeed, the athlete continued to consent to information about her disclosure and ongoing treatment to be appropriately shared, understanding the value of sharing this information in ensuring her continued support. One could argue that the psychologist's sensitive, early explanation that Amy's disclosure would need to be shared set the tone in this case study. However, even in cases where the individual asks for information not to be shared it is important that they understand the need for disclosures of this type to be shared appropriately in order to put the best support in place and to protect the mental health of the individual receiving the disclosure.

Conclusion

This case study demonstrates some of the support available to elite athletes in the UK and is an illustration of how a case can be appropriately managed in a collaborative way. It also emphasises the following key messages, which are relevant to all sports organisations:

- Disclosures about mental health concerns or the need to respond in a crisis could be experienced by anyone within a sport or team
- It is important that everyone knows the referral pathway within their particular sport or team and the wider support available
- Consider education which increases understanding of and comfort in talking about mental health, the benefits of an environment that promotes positive mental health and consideration of how to respond in a crisis
- Be aware of the 'ripple effects' on those involved in responding to or witnessing someone in crisis
- Consider how you can facilitate a shared understanding of someone who has experienced a mental health crisis in order to best-support them in their day-to-day life in elite sport

Glossary

CBT	Cognitive Behavioural Therapy
CHC	Culture Health Check
EIS	English Institute of Sport
HPS	High Performance System
MHEP	Mental Health Expert Panel
MHSG	Mental Health Steering Group
MHT	Mental Health Team
NGB	Sport's National Governing Body
TL	Technical Lead

References

Bathgate, F., Bennett, E., Cropper, J., Edwards, L., Emond, A., …, & Samuel, V. (2013). Good practice guidelines for clinical psychologists working in paediatric cochlear implant teams. *Cochlear Implants International 14*, 32–34. doi: 10.1179/1467010013Z.000000000131.

Bickley, J., Rogers, A., Bell, J., & Thombs, M. (2016). 'Elephant spotting': The importance of developing shared understanding to work more effectively with talented but challenging athletes. *Sport and Exercise Psychology Review 12*, 43–53.

British Psychological Society (2015). Special issue: Team formulation. *Clinical Psychology Forum* 275. Leicester, British Psychological Society.

Eynan, R., Bergmans, Y., Antony, J., Cutliffe, J. R., Harder, H. G., …, & Links, P. S. (2014). The effects of suicide ideation assessments on urges to self-harm and suicide. *Crisis 35*(2), 123–131.

Grey-Thompson, Baroness Tanni (2017, April). Duty of Care in Sport: Independent Report to Government. Retrieved from: https://assets.publishing.service.gov.uk/government/uploads/system/uploads/attachment_data/file/610130/Duty_of_Care_Review_-_April_2017__2.pdf.

Gould, M. S., Marrocco, F. A., Kleinman, M., Thomas, J. G., Mostkoff, K., …, & Davies, M. (2005). Evaluating iatrogenic risk of youth suicide screening programs. *Journal of the American Medical Association 293*(13), 1635–1643.

Iles, V., & Cranfield, S. (2004). Managing change in the NHS: Developing change management skills. London, UK: SDO. Retrieved from: www.netscc.ac.uk/netscc/hsdr/files/project/SDO_A1_08-1301-057_V01.pdf.

NCAA (2017, November) Summary of the Task Force to Advance Mental Health Best Practices. Retrieved from: www.ncaa.org/sport-science-institute/topics/summary-task-force-advance-mental-health-best-practices.

Northumberland, Tyne and Wear NHS Foundation Trust (2018). Understanding what influences your mental health and wellbeing. Retrieved from www.ntw.nhs.uk/content/uploads/2018/02/5-Ps-and-formulation-LP.pdf.

Portch (2019, December). Does your team take athlete engagement and wellbeing seriously enough? Retrieved from: https://leadersinsport.com/performance/ais-athlete-engagement-wellbeing/.

Reardon, C. L., Hainline, B., Aron, C. M., Baron, D., Baum, A. L., …, & Engebretsen, L. (2019) Mental health in elite athletes: International Olympic Committee consensus statement (2019). *British Journal of Sports Medicine 53,* 667–699. doi: 10.1136/bjsports-2019–100715.

UK Sport (2018). 2017 Culture Health Check Report. London, UK Sport. Retrieved from: www.uksport.gov.uk/~/media/files/chc-report-final.pdf?la=en.

11

FROM TRAGIC INCIDENTS TO SOUND VALUE-BASED LEADERSHIP

A summary

Carsten Hvid Larsen, Karin Moesch, Natalie Durand-Bush, and Kristoffer Henriksen

Winning "at any cost" is incompatible with a modern responsible sport system. Further, supporting mental health (MH) is a core component of any culture of excellence (Henriksen et al., 2019). But how do we go about it? MH support in elite sport is still in many ways treading virgin ground. As editors of this book, we are grateful to the authors who shared their MH experiences and work in their respective countries and outlined the lessons they learned. Below we briefly summarize key take home messages about MH in the form of five postulates.

We still do not quite grasp the nature of MH in elite sport

Many definitions of MH have been put forth across time and fields, and some are ill aligned with the nature of elite sport. We often unintentionally view MH as the absence of mental illness, which is most certainly an oversimplification. MH is a complex lived experience.

We generally support The World Health Organization's (WHO) definition of MH as "a state of well-being in which the individual realizes his or her own abilities, can cope with the normal stresses of life, can work productively and fruitfully, and is able to make a contribution to his or her community" (WHO, 2014). This definition of MH adopts a positive psychology perspective and represents a more holistic view, emphasizing well-being as a core construct. However, we also issue a word of caution as this definition raises concerns and lends itself to potential misunderstandings as it identifies positive feelings and positive functioning as key factors for MH, and does not account for specific contextual factors. Periodic experiences of unpleasant thoughts and emotions, such as performance anxiety, are a natural part of athletic pursuits and should not be pathologized.

We want to highlight the need for sport organizations to discuss and explicitly define what they mean by MH as part of their efforts to build systems that support it. In some of the chapters, for example Canada, such discussions were deemed essential for the development of effective mental health services. MH definitions should be inclusive and take into consideration the context. Galderisi et al.'s (2015) definition of MH integrates sociocultural factors and values; however, it is not sport-specific. Additional work is warranted to establish a comprehensive MH definition for elite sport.

The initiation of MH programs should not have to rely on tragic incidents

What does it take for sport organizations to take MH seriously? A media scandal? A tragic suicide? It is indicated in some chapters how a tragic incident (e.g., a suicide) was instrumental in the initiation of a national MH program. Some authors even describe a "need" for a tragic incident in the country before organizations sound the alarm bell and start developing proper programs. This was, for example, the case in Germany, where the tragic suicide of a national football goalkeeper stimulated the development of a system to prevent MH tragedies from happening again.

In some chapters, the authors portray a national awareness of MH problems in their country alongside tragic and publicly known incidents, which are not followed by the initiation of national programs or clinics. What leads these countries to omit establishing structures to oversee MH when the need is clearly there? Certainly, some factors include the economy and sport system in these particular countries; setting up MH support systems is unquestionably costly. Another factor seems to be the tradition for sport psychology in certain countries. MH is often considered a natural extension of the sport psychology field and sport psychology practitioners are expected to play a key role in the area. But sport psychology can be an underdeveloped area compared to other expert areas (e.g., physiology and medicine). Sport psychology may also yet have to establish itself as a worthwhile endeavor for elite athletes in some countries. This was the case in Brazil and Taiwan, where sport psychology had a strong tradition to focus solely on performance. If managers, coaches, and athletes hold negative attitudes toward sport psychology, this implicitly affects their attitudes toward mental health services.

Fortunately, some chapters highlight that after programmes are developed, there seems to be a positive tendency toward the de-stigmatization of MH problems in sport. As the programs are established and grow in recognition, more and more stakeholders in the field of elite sport understand that MH disorders such as depression, anxiety, and eating disorders naturally occur in sport and life, and are not a sign of weakness. They acknowledge that action must be taken to prevent, address, or treat such disorders. The battle for MH support in elite sport should be promoted and destigmatized through information and enlightenment, in line with sound values rather than tragic incidents.

Mental health is deeply contextualized

As alluded to above in our discussion of definitions, how MH is understood and fostered varies depending on contexts. Individual (e.g., race and gender), environment (e.g., national, political, and sport-specific) and developmental (e.g., age and career phase) contexts all shape lived experiences of MH. The current book provides unique insights into how MH is conceived and dealt with in different countries. It is clear that to arrive at a contextualized understanding of MH, it is important to take into consideration the impact of social and economic MH determinants in a particular country. When we compare the chapter describing MH in sub-Saharan Africa with that addressing MH in western Europe, Canada, and Australia, there are significant differences regarding definitions, attitudes, and priorities surrounding MH and the general field of sport psychology. On the one hand, the examples from Germany, England, Australia, Sweden, and Canada illustrate systems with commitment and dedicated resources for the prevention of MH challenges and the promotion of thriving and the retention of athletes. On the other hand, the chapter from the African continent describes how MH and sport psychology, in general, receive very little attention from policy makers and governments, which is closely related to the reality of general social welfare in African countries.

MH is further related to national culture and religion. In sub-Saharan Africa, the authors provide insightful accounts of the strong influence of political corruption in elite sport and indigenous culture in sport psychology practice. Many people in Africa strongly believe that mental illness is caused by and can be treated through traditional and supernatural powers. In Brazil, a country with overwhelming socioeconomic challenges, a lack of adequate nutrition and basic facilities in some youth academies take precedence over MH services in terms of focus and financial priority. In Taiwan, potential monetary rewards for sport success present unique MH challenges, fueling the "win at all cost" mentality.

These complexities require deep cultural competence. We need to truly understand and consider the culture and context when conceptualizing MH, building national support systems, and providing MH services in different countries. Special care must also be taken to adapt diagnosis and treatment tools developed in Western countries for effective use in countries with very different cultures.

There is no "one size fits all" approach to organizing MH services across countries

In our view, a focus on MH is key in any sound sport system, and sport organizations have a responsibility to create elite sport environments that support athlete MH. Such systems should provide the structures and resources to promote positive MH by cultivating help-seeking, by building MH literacy, and by providing athletes opportunities to develop psychological skills, and prevent mental disorders through early identification and treatment of symptoms. We recognize, however, that the systems set in place to support athlete MH worldwide must and will vary to account for cultural and organizational differences. Looking across the chapters in the book, we find examples of different approaches to MH across the different countries. From a macro perspective, differences are found in overall national structures and MH programs. From a micro perspective, differences are found in specific intervention methods, local programming, and ways that clinics are run.

Several chapters describe how leading sport organizations (e.g., NGBs, Olympic committees) play a key role in addressing MH. In Canada, the authors describe how informing and mobilizing key stakeholders and organizations were necessary for the implementation of services and resources to promote MH, prevent mental illness, and provide appropriate care to Canadian high-performance athletes experiencing MH challenges. In Canada, establishing a collaborative model of care was recognized as the gold standard to effectively address MH and disorders and thus became the essence of the national structure (i.e., Canadian Centre for Mental Health and Sport). In Germany, the initiatives *mentaltalent* and *MentalEmpowerment* are tasked with systematically structuring and providing sport psychology services in order to promote MH. If athletes require referral to psychotherapeutic or psychiatric care, *MentalEmpowerment* provides contact to specialized experts and therapy. A host of professions successfully collaborate to provide holistic care in Germany, and yet the authors highlight potential future improvements including a positive climate around cooperation among different health care professionals (sport psychologists, psychiatrists and psychotherapists). In Sweden, national clinics are based on a unique collaboration between sport governing bodies and the public health care system, leading to the establishment of important knowledge hubs for MH in elite sport. A very different picture is seen in Brazil, where neither the major sport organizations nor the national health care systems seem to have a dedicated focus on athlete MH.

Looking beyond overall national structures to zero in on the implementation of MH services, it is clear that service provision programs and protocols should consider several important factors. These include but are not limited to:

- The purpose of the clinic or program and targeted population (e.g., elite athletes, coaches, support staff);
- The coordination of multidisciplinary staff (e.g., psychiatrists, clinical psychologists, sport psychologists, or other relevant experts) regarding diagnoses and treatment plans;
- Eligibility criteria as well as intake and assessment tools and procedures (e.g., intake interview, self-report questionnaires, biomarkers, functional behavioral analysis);
- Treatment approaches (e.g., CBT, ACT);
- Protocols for informing and involving coaches and sport staff (e.g., athletic trainers, nutritionists);
- Contextual knowledge of the elite sport environment of all staff involved in the service provision programs.

Differences in MH service provision between countries are evident. In Australia, an effort to build closer relationships between the Australian Institute of Sport MH team and national sporting organizations has facilitated increased understanding, communication, and collaboration. This has led to the clarification of athlete MH needs and the establishment of different practitioner roles for supporting athletes. In Sweden and Canada, athletes and coaches can seek help directly from the national clinics/centre and do not require an external referral. Practitioners have knowledge of the elite sport context, leading them to provide comprehensive sport-centered care. In the case of Taiwan, the lack of protocols made the MH of athlete dependent on the coach, who himself was challenged by long working hours and little time for recovery. Examples of MH services in the chapters also pinpoint the need to move beyond service provision in the form of treatment to take a more proactive and preventative approach to maximize and maintain well-being. For example, in the US, practitioners adopt approaches such as Acceptance Commitment Therapy to not only reduce mental illness symptoms (e.g., health anxiety) but also enrich athletic performance to enable athletes to live a fulfilling and meaningful life, even in the face of MH challenges.

Leadership is key to securing MH resources and athlete retention

In two multi-societal consensus statements on athlete MH, Henriksen and colleagues (2019; 2020) advocate the need for clear MH leadership and a MH officer (MHO). The main functions of a MHO are to support athlete MH, which includes designing, implementing, and evaluating a structure or system for MH promotion and mental illness prevention and treatment.

This system should address assessment and relevance of MH components, and adherence to professional, ethical, and moral service delivery standards (Henriksen et al., 2019). A focus on MH transcends athletic achievement thus it is suggested that the MHO should be someone who is not responsible for athletic performance.

Across the established programmes and services described in this book, the need for leadership and management of MH within any given country and sport system is evident. For instance, the Swedish, Canadian, Australian, English, and German initiatives were all dependent on clear leadership and resource mobilization. In a similar vein, we also see how an absence of leadership and organizational back-up can be a barrier to successful MH service provision. This was well illustrated in the chapter addressing the situation in Brazil. However, we need not look to socioeconomically challenged countries to see such manifestations. For example, Denmark, a western European country with a solid welfare system, has yet to develop a systematic approach to athlete MH with dedicated leadership.

Based on the examples presented in this book, we advocate that to successfully address MH in any elite sport system, leadership must be engaged at all levels and specifically assigned stakeholders within major sport organizations (e.g., each NGB, Olympic Committee) must make MH their primary focus. Whether in the shape of a MHO or a collaborative MH team, leaders should focus on supporting athletes to live meaningful lives regardless of their podium status. They should also equip them to thrive and succeed despite experiencing mental health difficulties, which is likely inevitable at some point in their athletic career. Michael Phelps serves as an important reminder that achieving the highest level in Olympic sport is possible despite battling mental illness (Champions Unplugged, 2018). Such committed leadership actions will likely improve the retention of athletes and inspire some of them to become MH ambassadors in their sport. This may have a positive impact on the broader culture surrounding MH in a particular country, leading to much needed stigma reduction and increased help-seeking.

References

Champions Unplugged (2018, October). Retrieved from: https://championsunplugged.com/2018/05/.

Galderisi, S., Heinz, A., Kastrup, M., Beezhold, J., & Sartorius, N. (2015). Toward a new definition of mental health. World Psychiatry *14*(2), 231–233. doi: 10.1002/wps.20231.

Henriksen, K., Schinke, R. J., McCann, S., Durand-Bush, N., Moesch, K., Parham, WD., Larsen, C. H., Cogan, K., Donaldsen, A., Poczwardowski, A., Noce, F., & Hunziker, J. (2020). Athlete mental health in the Olympic/Paralympic quadrennium: A multi-societal consensus statement. *International Journal of Sport and Exercise Psychology 18*, 391–408.

Henriksen, K., Schinke R. J., Moesch, K., McCann, S., Parham W. D., Larsen, C. H., & Terry, P. (2019). Consensus statement on improving the mental health of high-performance athletes. *International Journal of Sport and Exercise Psychology 18*(5), 553–560. https://doi.org/10.1080/1612197X.2019.1570473

World Health Organization (WHO). (2014). *Mental health: A state of well-being*. Geneva, Switzerland: World Health Organization.

INDEX

For Product Safety Concerns and Information please contact our EU
representative GPSR@taylorandfrancis.com
Taylor & Francis Verlag GmbH, Kaufingerstraße 24, 80331 München, Germany

www.ingramcontent.com/pod-product-compliance
Ingram Content Group UK Ltd.
Pitfield, Milton Keynes, MK11 3LW, UK
UKHW052211190926
475702UK00006B/969
* 9 7 8 0 3 6 7 4 2 7 6 7 2 *